Diet, Lipoproteins and Coronary Heart Disease

A biochemical perspective

EH Mangiapane
AM Salter

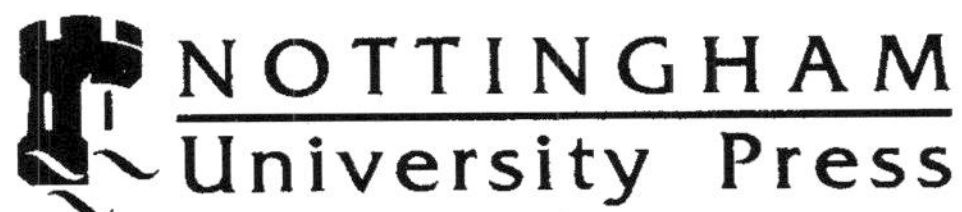

Nottingham University Press
Manor Farm, Main Street, Thrumpton
Nottingham, NG11 0AX, United Kingdom

NOTTINGHAM

First published 1999
Reprinted 2001

British Library Cataloguing in Publication Data
Diet, Lipoproteins and Coronary Heart Disease: A biochemical perspective
Mangiapane, EH
Salter, AM

ISBN 1-897676-81-6

Typeset by Nottingham University Press, Nottingham
Printed and bound by The Cromwell Press, Trowbridge, Wiltshire

CONTENTS

1 Coronary Heart Disease: an overview

1.1 Introduction

While death is inevitable, cause of death and life expectancy varies enormously depending on where we live, who we are and, in many cases, what we do or do not eat. For the majority of people in the world the major problem is still the availability of enough food to provide sufficient energy to sustain life and the appropriate concentrations of essential nutrients to maintain normal bodily functions. On the other hand, in many of the "developed" countries "over-nutrition" is the major problem associated with the diet. Cardiovascular disease, cancer, obesity and diabetes represent the main health problems of most industrialised nations. Each of these chronic diseases is related to diet.

1.2 Diet, morbidity and mortality

Humans evolved as omnivores, able to survive on diets in which either animal or plant tissues predominate. Even in the world today examples can be found of these two extremes. Our earliest ancestors were "hunter-gatherers" and, at least in fertile areas, this was likely to provide a varied diet. Consideration of analogous populations that still survive today show a lower fat intake and a greater unsaturated to saturated fatty acid ratio than in the diets of developed countries. In addition, our ancestors consumed substantially more fibre. However, such a dependence on "wild" food obviously meant that humans were at the mercy of the environment and famine and diseases related to poor nutrition must have been common. The development of agriculture considerably improved the consistency of food availability in many parts of the world. Coupled with the development of industry (and the wealth it created) and vast improvements in public health, these changes in lifestyle have dramatically changed the patterns of disease and considerably extended our expected life span. Figure 1.1 shows the changes in life expectancy in the developed and developing world. The large gap between the rich and poor nations is predicted to close rapidly into the next century. There is also a considerable difference in the causes of death between these two populations (figure 1.2). In the developing world, in 1980, infectious and parasitic disease accounted for 40% of all deaths while only 8% of people died from such causes in the developed world. In contrast, 54% of people died from cardiovascular disease in developed countries compared to only 19% in the emerging nations.

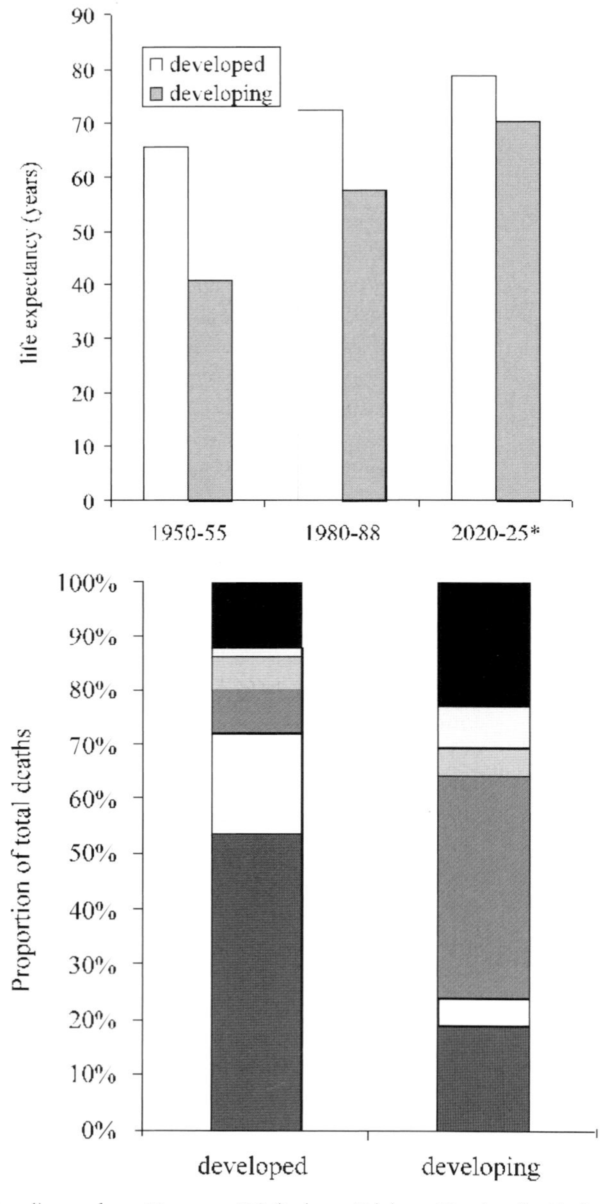

Figure 1.1
Life expectancy in the developed and developing world. Data from Diet, Nutrition and the Prevention of chronic disease (WHO, Technical Report series 797). *predicted value

Figure 1.2
Causes of death in the developed and developing world. Data for 1980 taken from Diet, Nutrition and the Prevention of chronic disease (WHO, Technical Report series 797)

This changing pattern of morbidity and mortality is probably due to a number of factors. First of all the very fact that we are living for longer has changed the pattern of disease. Cardiovascular disease is a chronic problem that develops over many years. Thus, in populations where life expectancy due to other diseases is often less than 60 years, it is unlikely that cardiovascular disease will be a major problem. As life span has increased we have begun to see increases in the incidence of chronic disease such as cardiovascular disease. Public health and medical developments have also made a major impact on causes of illness and death. Many infectious diseases have been virtually eradicated from the developed world and many of those remaining are no longer life threatening. Finally, lifestyle changes have contributed to the changes in pattern of disease with diet representing one of the most important aspects. In many Western countries it is not unusual to consume over 50% of total energy intake as fat with a high proportion consisting of saturated fatty acids. High intakes of energy-dense fat coupled with a sedentary lifestyle frequently leads to obesity. Obesity is frequently associated with non-insulin dependent diabetes and both conditions are linked with an increased risk of developing cardiovascular disease. Furthermore, as will be discussed in chapter 7, high saturated fatty acid intakes are associated with elevated plasma cholesterol concentration. Diets rich in saturated fatty acids are also associated with certain types of cancer. Thus, over a relatively short period of time, too short to see any biological evolution, our diet has evolved dramatically compared to our "hunter-gatherer" ancestors. It is hardly surprising that this has resulted in major changes the causes of morbidity and mortality.

1.3 Cardiovascular disease and the clinical manifestations of atherosclerosis

As described above, a major cause of death in the developed countries is cardiovascular disease, which arises from the development of atherosclerosis in certain arteries. The changes, which occur in the artery wall in atherosclerosis, are described in chapter 2. Below are discussed the main clinical manifestations of atherosclerosis: coronary artery disease, atherosclerotic cerebral vascular disease and peripheral arterial disease.

Coronary heart disease

The main supply of oxygen to heart muscle is *via* the coronary arteries (figure 1.3). When insufficient oxygen reaches the heart muscle, or myocardium, ischemia results. **Myocardial ischemia** can occur if the lumen of a coronary artery is narrowed by an atheromatous plaque or if the plaque fissures and becomes the site of a thrombus formation, thus obscuring the flow of blood through the vessel.

Myocardial ischemia can also occur from other diseases, such as cardiovascular syphilis and rheumatic heart disease. The term **coronary heart disease** (CHD) is used here to refer to cardiac disease due specifically to atherosclerosis of the coronary arteries.

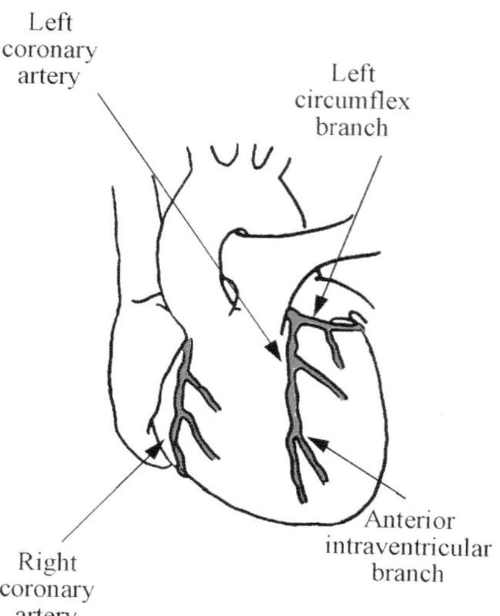

Figure 1.3
The coronary arteries

Myocardial ischemia can give rise to **angina pectoris**. In this condition there is a dull discomfort in the substernal area and pain may be felt in the upper epigastrium, and may radiate to the neck and down one or both arms. The symptoms, which appear with exertion, excitement or distress disappear with removal of the stress which induced the pain. As chest pains are not necessarily the result of angina, examining an electrocardiogram assists diagnosis. Changes of the latter occur if myocardial ischemia persists.

Myocardial infarction, commonly known as a "heart attack", results when prolonged ischemia leads to necrosis or cell death of heart muscle cells. The major symptom of a myocardial infarct is substernal discomfort, which feels like a crushing weight upon the chest. Pain radiates into the neck and arms. This pain, if untreated and if the patient survives, may persist for a few hours or even days. Confirmation of a diagnosis is assisted by characteristic electrocardium traces and changes of serum enzyme levels. Sudden ischemia of the myocardium can be the cause of **sudden death** where an apparently healthy individual suddenly collapses and dies.

Atherosclerotic cerebral vascular disease

Thrombosis of cerebral vessels is the most common form of disease producing cerebral vascular accident but it may be difficult to distinguish between this and cerebral embolism, intracerebral hemorrhage, subarachnoid hemorrhage and short term ischemia. Intracerebral hemorrhage, caused by rupture of an intracranial artery, and subarachnoid hemorrhage, caused by rupture of an aneurism in the Circle of Willis, are both accompanied by blood in the cerebrospinal fluid.

Atheroma in arteries in the brain can restrict blood flow and produce transient ischemia. Sufficient narrowing produced by the atheroma alone, or a thrombus formed on an ulcerating atheroma, can lead to more profound ischemia and cause **cerebral infarction or stroke**. The symptoms of the stroke are dependent upon the size of the region rendered ischemic and its location in the brain. Strokes may also result from cerebral embolism: emboli from atheromatous lesions outside the brain may travel in the blood and subsequently occlude cerebral vessels.

Peripheral arterial disease

Atherosclerosis in the arteries of the lower extremities, in the aorta, the femoral, the iliac and popliteal arteries can cause narrowing of the arteries and attendant ischemia of the tissues supplied by these arteries. The symptoms of **intermittent claudication** are characterised by pain in the calf muscles after walking. The pain is relieved when the muscles are inactive, i.e. when the patient stops walking. Severe ischemia may result in gangrene of the extremities.

Prevalence of atherosclerotic disease

The prevalence of the three forms of atherosclerotic disease has been determined in a number of epidemiological studies. Perhaps the most famous of these is the Framingham study. The results of this study, relating to the incidence of coronary heart disease, cerebral vascular disease and peripheral artery disease in a population in America, are shown in table 1.1.

The problem of a high incidence of premature death due to cardiovascular disease in England was recognised in the Government White Paper "Health of the Nation" in 1992. This set targets for reducing coronary heart disease and stroke deaths as outlined in table 1.2.

1.4 Conclusion

The high incidence of death due to cardiovascular diseases in developed countries and, as their economies and lifestyles change, the increasing problem these disease pose to the developing world, make it critical that we continue to try and understand the aetiology of these diseases. In the chapters, which follow, we will explain how our diet influences the development of cardiovascular disease and discuss possible ways of reducing the incidence of death from atherosclerosis-related diseases, in particular coronary heart disease.

Data from the Framingham Study: in this study 5127 men and women living in the town of Framingham, in USA, were observed by clinicians for 24 years.

Table 1.1 Clinical manifestations of atherosclerosis

Number of subjects who developed:	*Men*	*Women*
Coronary heart disease		
Angina Pectoris	277	243
Total myocardial infarction	365	155
Myocardial infarction revealed by electrocardiogram	301	121
Coronary insufficiency	71	53
Sudden death attributed to coronary heart disease	130	43
Death, not sudden, attributed to coronary heart disease	150	75
Cerebral vascular accident		
Atherothrombotic brain infarction	94	105
Cerebral embolism	23	25
Peripheral arterial disease		
Intermittent claudication	155	103
Total	1566	923

Table 1.2 "Health of the Nation" targets for reduction of coronary heart disease and stroke

Age group	*Disease*	*1990*	*2000 (target)*
		deaths per 100,000	
Under 65	CHD	58	35
	Stroke	12.5	7.5
65-74	CHD	899	629
	Stroke	No target	

2 Atherosclerosis

2.1 Introduction

Atherosclerosis is a disease in which the structure of certain arteries is altered by formation of atheroma in the artery wall. The development of atheroma will be discussed below. The clinical symptoms of atherosclerosis include myocardial infarction (heart attack) and stroke. These dreadful and often fatal consequences of atherosclerosis have led to the research into the development and progression of atherosclerosis and the possibilities of treatment and regression of atherosclerosis before life threatening conditions are reached.

The term arteriosclerosis was introduced in 1829 to describe the scarring and calcification seen in post mortem arteries. The term atherosclerosis, used first in 1904, was employed to describe lipid rich deposits seen in arteriosclerosis. The link between the clinical symptoms and signs of myocardial infarction and atherosclerosis and thrombosis of the coronary arteries was made by James Herrick in 1912.

Atherosclerosis begins in childhood but clinical manifestations may not occur until late adulthood. Lipids can accumulate in the intima of large elastic and muscular arteries. Initially lipid deposits are known as **fatty streaks**. At some sites in the coronary arteries, in the aorta, in the cerebral arteries or the iliac and femoral arteries, fatty streaks thicken by continuous, or intermittent, accumulation of lipid and connective tissue to form **fibrous plaques** or **atheroma**. These atheroma gradually increase in size and can undergo calcification and vascularisation. They can then haemorrhage or ulcerate and consequently become sites for the formation of thrombi, i.e. blood clots. Advanced atherosclerotic lesions, in the absence or presence of adhering thrombi, can occlude arteries, reduce blood supply to tissues and produce severe clinical symptoms. Thrombi that become detached from the vessel wall are termed **emboli** and these may occlude distal vessels and also produce clinical symptoms.

A diagram showing the main arteries arising from the aorta is shown in figure 2.1. Lesions may be found in the human aorta in the first decade, in the coronary arteries in the second decade and in cerebral arteries in the third and fourth decades of life. Clinically manifest coronary heart disease and peripheral vascular disease usually occur in the fifth decade and stroke in the sixth decade of life or later.

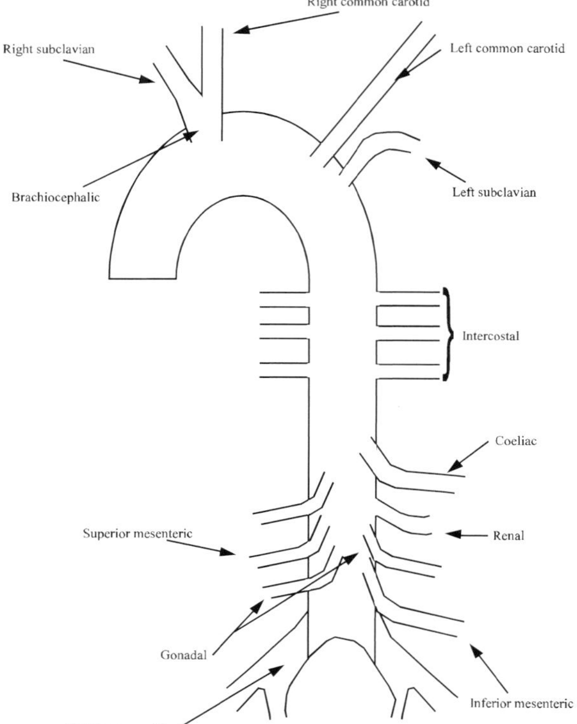

Figure 2.1
Main arteries arising from the aorta

2.2 Methods of investigation of atherosclerosis

Human studies

As described above atherosclerosis, in man, may take many years, to develop to the point where clinical symptoms are evident. It is not generally possible to determine the early stages of atherosclerosis in humans, at least while they are alive, because the atherosclerotic lesions usually occur in vital arteries. Studies of the early stages of lesion development, therefore, are confined to post-mortem measurements. Once clinical symptoms are present, which usually means that atherosclerosis is well advanced, there are a number of methods available to examine lesions that have already formed. **Angiography** involves injecting an opaque dye into the blood stream and taking x-rays of the vascular system. This technique will show which vessels are affected by atherosclerosis if the latter produces a significant narrowing of the artery lumen. However, this is an invasive technique that is not free of risk. There is the risk of exposure to x-rays and possible reaction to the contrast medium. **Intravascular ultrasound**, which permits a three dimensional examination of the artery lumen, is also invasive as a microphone has to be placed in the vessel to be examined. A non-invasive method that is currently being investigated is **magnetic resonance imaging (MRI)**.

Animal studies

Animal studies have made a major contribution to our understanding of the development of atherosclerosis. A wide variety of species have been used in such studies but some caution must be shown in the interpretation of animal experiments due to the major differences in lipoprotein metabolism between man and many other species. A number of species of primate including rhesus monkey, African green monkey and cynomologous monkey have proved useful in the study of lipoprotein metabolism and atherosclerosis, but both ethical and economic reasons have prevented the widespread use of primates.

One of the most widely used animal models of atherosclerosis is the rabbit. Cholesterol feeding in this species leads to massive accumulation of cholesterol in the plasma and the development of extensive lipid deposits in the arteries. However, this hypercholesterolaemia is associated with the accumulation of a specific lipoprotein class (β - very low-density lipoprotein) which does not normally occur in humans. Another problem has been the considerable variation between animals in plasma lipids and extent of atherosclerosis. One rabbit model however, the Watanabe heritable hyperlipidaemic (WHHL) rabbit, has been found to exhibit the same gene defect as humans suffering from familial hypercholesterolaemia. Understanding of this disease, which results from a deficiency of functional low density lipoprotein (LDL) receptors (see chapter 5), and it's association with atherosclerosis, has been dramatically improved by the study of the WHHL rabbit.

Other species that develop atherosclerotic lesions include the pig, hamster and pigeon.

The most recent animals to be used extensively in atherosclerosis research are mice. While many strains of mouse are resistant to the development of atherosclerotic lesions a number of inbred strains have been found which do develop fairly discreet lesions in response to a high saturated fat, high cholesterol diet. However, much more widespread and advanced lesions have been found in genetically modified and transgenic mice. The best studied so far are the LDL receptor and apolipoprotein E knockout mice (see chapter 5). Such technology is being used to investigate a wide range of influences on lipoprotein metabolism and atherogenesis.

Cell culture

Aortic endothelial cells may be grown in culture. So too can isolated aortic smooth muscle cells. Much has been learned about the biochemistry of these cells from these cell culture systems. A co-culture of endothelial cells grown over a layer of aortic smooth muscle cells has been described, which is a more appropriate system to investigate events that might operate *in vivo*, in the intact artery wall, where there is interaction between the different types of cells in the intima. Studies on isolated aortic cells in culture and co-culture are discussed in chapter 6.

2.3 The normal artery wall

Structure of the normal artery wall

Diagrams of the structure of the artery wall are shown in figure 2.2.

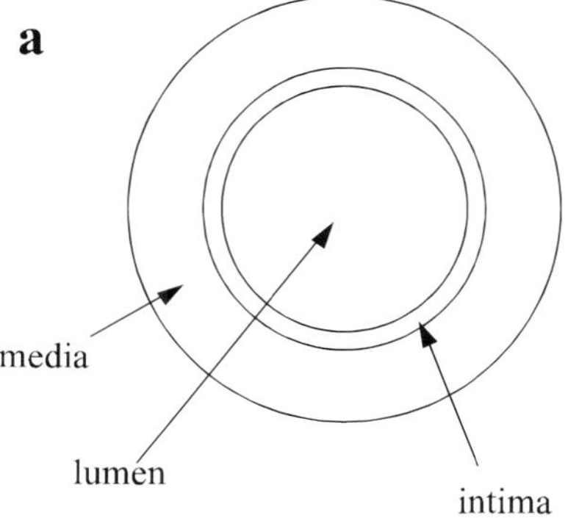

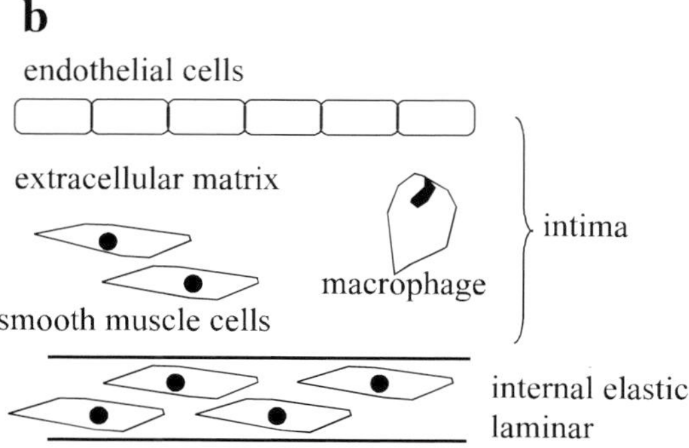

Figure 2.2 Structure of the artery wall

a) Cross section of the artery
b) Intimal region of the artery wall

Endothelial cells form a continuous monolayer on the surface of the artery wall, acting as a boundary between the artery lumen and the artery wall. The endothelial cells and the subendothelial space, between the endothelial cells and the media is known as the **intima**; it comprises the endothelial cells, connective tissue, a few smooth muscle-like cells, called the myointimal cells, and isolated macrophages. The **internal elastic lamina** is the boundary between the intima and the underlying media, but this may be absent in some parts of the artery. In elastic arteries, e.g. the aorta, subclavian and carotid arteries, the intima lies above the **tunica media** that comprises interspersed layers of elastic tissue and smooth muscle. In muscular arteries e.g. the coronary and femoral arteries, the intima is separated from the underlying muscular tunica media by a discrete internal elastic lamina. The intima itself comprises two regions: beneath the endothelial cells is the **proteoglycan layer** which contains, non -fibrous connective tissue, the proteoglycan ground substance, and few elastic fibres. **Smooth muscle cells**, exhibiting two distinct phenotypes are also present. The synthetic phenotype, are rich in rough endoplasmic reticulum while the contractile phenotype are rich in myofibrils. In addition, isolated **macrophages** are present. Below this proteoglycan layer is the **musculoelastic layer** in which there are many smooth muscle cells of the contractile phenotype and elastic fibres and collagen are in abundance.

The **extracellular matrix**, which comprises up to 60% of the volume of the intima, contains molecules synthesised and secreted by both endothelial and smooth muscle cells. Underlying the endothelial cells are **proteoglycans** which comprise mainly chondroitin sulphate and dermatan sulphate proteoglycans (see below). These molecules interact with other matrix proteins such as collagens, elastin and fibronectin. In normal human coronary arteries the content of these proteoglycans increases with age but also increases in atherosclerosis.

Proteoglycans contain a core protein to which one or more glycosaminoglycans are covalently attached through O-glycosidic linkages to serine residues in the protein. In addition to the glycosaminoglycans both N- and O- linked oligosaccharides may be present. **Chondroitin sulphate proteoglycan** (also known as versecan) is a large molecule whose protein core is 263kD with 15-20 glycosoaminoglycan chains attached; comprising 70% chondroitin 6 sulphate, 20% chondroitin 4 sulphate and 10% dermatan sulphate. Chondroitin sulphate proteoglycan forms a three dimensional network with hyaluronate giving the intima its strength and ability to be compressed. **Dermatan sulphate proteoglycan** has a smaller core protein, and 2-3 glycosaminoglycan side chains; the dermatan sulphate proteoglycans known as decorin and biglycan have a core protein of 36kD and 2-3 side chains of dermatan sulphate and function to maintain the orientation of collagen fibres in the intima. The proteoglycan, perlecan, is associated with the basement membrane found beneath the endothelial cells; this proteoglycan comprises a core protein of 450kD and 3 heparin sulphate chains which bind collagen, vitronectin and laminin and thus this proteoglycan is involved in anchoring endothelial cells to the basement membrane. Endothelial cells synthesise and secrete heparin sulphate- and dermatin sulphate- containing proteoglycans. The former is found on the cell surface and in the basement membrane of endothelial cells. Smooth muscle cells synthesise and secrete chondroitin sulphate-, dermatan sulphate- and to a lesser extent heparin sulphate-proteoglycans. Macrophages synthesise and secrete chondroitin sulphate proteoglycan and heparin sulphate proteoglycan.

The major types of **collagen** in the arterial intima are types I and III. Type III is found in the subendothelial region of the intima and is probably synthesised by endothelial cells. Type I collagen in the intima increases with age and this may reflect an increased synthesis by smooth muscle cells in the intima.

Elastic fibres are particularly found in the musculoelastic region of the intima. The precursor of the **elastin** component of elastic fibres is tropoelastin that is secreted from intimal cells: both endothelial cells and smooth muscle cells can synthesise this protein.

Fibronectin is a high molecular weight glycoprotein found on cell surfaces, in extracellular matrix and in the blood. It has a collagen binding domain and can also bind heparin and thus it helps bind cells to the extracellular matrix. **Laminin** is also an extracellular glycoprotein: this is a major component of the basement membrane underlying the endothelium.

Adaptive intimal thickening

Physiological adaptation to changes in pulse rate, blood pressure, arterial geometry, flow rate, resistance to flow in distal vessels and organs, results in **adaptive intimal thickening**. The latter is of two types: **eccentric intimal thickening** and **diffuse intimal thickening**. These are characterised by thickened intima and by a higher turnover of endothelial and smooth muscle cells and an increased concentration of plasma lipoprotein. It should be noted that adaptive intimal thickening is a normal physiological response and not a pathological change.

Eccentric intimal thickening is a focal thickening located on the outer walls opposite the flow divider of a bifurcation, where a single vessel divides into two or where a branch leaves the main vessel (see figure 2.3). It extends for a short distance along the length of the artery proximal and distal to the flow divider. This type of intimal thickening is seen in the coronary, carotid, cerebral and renal arteries. The extent of diffuse intimal thickening is not certain.

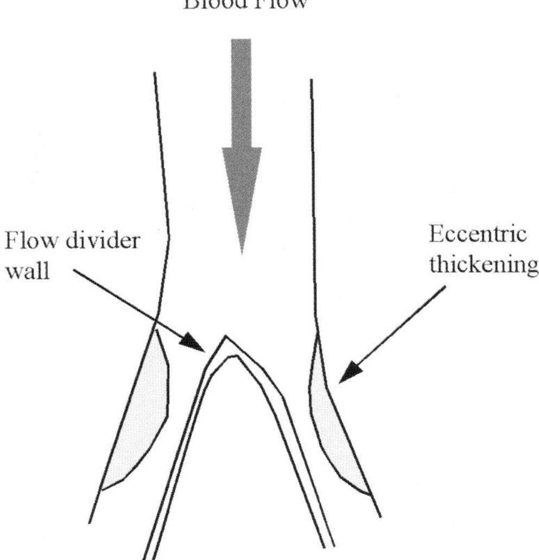

Figure 2.3
Eccentric intimal thickening

As described earlier, two types of smooth muscle cells are found in the intima as described above. An increase in smooth muscle cells in the intima during adaptive intimal thickening may occur by division of cells already present within the intima or by transmigration of cells from the media.

Advanced atherosclerotic lesions are frequently observed to occur earlier in adaptive intimal thickening than in thinner regions of intima. However, in severe atherosclerosis, advanced lesions are not confined to the regions of adaptive thickening.

Physiological properties of the artery wall

Endothelial cells

Endothelial cells of normal arteries are flattened, elongated, polygonal cells with the long axes generally oriented in the direction of blood flow. Endothelial cells contain normal organelles and a cytoskeleton of microfilaments, microtubules and intermediate filaments. They also contain a large number of plasmalemmal vesicles involved in transcytosis (transport of macromolecules across the cell) and, characteristic of endothelial cells, Weibel-Palade bodies, rod shaped bodies containing factor VIII related antigen and von Willebrand factor. Endothelial cells have a variety of physiological functions in the normal artery wall. These include the following:

1. Action as a permeability barrier.

   There is traffic of plasma proteins and lipoproteins across normal endothelium. Transport across the endothelium can occur by transcytosis, in plasmalemmal vesicles, and through intercellular junctions. The rate of transport depends upon the plasma concentration, the size and charge of the proteins or particles, the location of the endothelium, and the age and blood pressure of the individual.

On the luminal surface, the endothelial cells are covered in a glycocalyx containing polysacharides, glycosaminoglycans and glycoproteins. Some of the latter bind lectins or proteoglycans such as heparin sulphate. The endothelial cell surface also has receptors for native LDL, insulin and histamine.

2. Provision of a non-thrombogenic surface and a surface to which few cells normally adhere.

   Normally the endothelium does not support the adherence of platelets or leukocytes and thrombi do not form on normal endothelium. The endothelial cell membrane contains thrombomodulin, which binds thrombin, and prevents clot formation.

3. Maintenance of basement membrane collagen and proteoglycans.

   Endothelial cells synthesise and secrete extracellular matrix components such as fibronectin, and components of the endothelial cell basement membrane: type IV and type V collagen, laminin and proteoglycans.

4. Maintenance of vascular tone by release of prostacyclin, nitric oxide and endothelin.

   Endothelial cells and smooth muscle cells synthesise and secrete prostacyclin, which inhibits platelet aggregation and causes vascular relaxation. Another vasodilator produced by endothelial cells is nitric oxide, which acts on the guanylate cyclase of smooth muscle cells. Nitric oxide also inhibits platelet aggregation. Endothelial cells may also stimulate vasoconstriction through production of endothelin, a peptide of 21 amino acids, which activates calcium channels in smooth muscle cells and stimulates contraction of myofibrils in these cells.

5. Formation and secretion of growth regulatory molecules and cytokines.

   An early event in atherogenesis, i.e. the development of atherosclerosis, may be endothelial cell injury, not physical injury as such, but endothelial dysfunction. Changes to one or more of the above functions may lead to endothelial dysfunction that could promote or facilitate the development of atherosclerosis. From studies of human tissue and of animals with atherosclerotic lesions there is evidence that the endothelium is not physically damaged in early atherosclerotic lesions but endothelial cells in these lesions may have a higher rate of turnover, and an increased permeability to macromolecules compared to normal endothelium. There may be impairment of endothelial dependent vasodilation and a stimulation of endothelial dependent vasoconstriction. The biochemical changes that accompany changes in endothelial function during the development of atherosclerosis will be discussed in chapter 6.

Smooth muscle cells

The role of smooth muscle cells in normal intima is uncertain. Many biochemical, physiological and pharmacological studies have been carried out on vascular smooth muscle cells in culture. However, it is likely that in most of these studies, where arteries provided the cells, that the smooth muscle cells derived from both the intima and the underlying media of the artery wall. Hence it is difficult to ascribe a precise function to the specifically intimal smooth muscle cells. In addition, in atheromatous lesions, where the number of smooth muscle cells increase compared with normal intima, these cells appear to be derived from proliferation of both intimal smooth muscle cells and medial smooth muscle cells which migrate into the intima.

The following functions have been attributed to smooth muscle cells, mainly from the *in vitro* studies. These functions may occur in normal intima but probably assume greater importance in atherosclerosis.

1. Synthesis of extracellular matrix components.

   Smooth muscle cells can synthesise collagen, elastin and proteoglycans as described above and thus contribute to neointimal growth. The latter occurs in developing atherosclerotic lesions and in the restenosis (re-blockage) that may occur after surgery to clear stenosed (blocked) coronary arteries. This surgical technique is known as angioplasty.

2. Ability to proliferate.

   Smooth muscle cells express various growth factor receptors and will proliferate in response to these growth factors. The latter may be released during injury of the endothelium, such as may occur during surgery, or may accumulate when the functions of the endothelium are impaired as occurs in atherosclerosis.

3. Removal of lipoproteins.

   The smooth muscle cells have plasma membrane LDL receptors so that the cells can obtain cholesterol from LDL in normal intima. During atherogenesis this normal function may be enhanced as these cells can accumulate lipid and become foam cells.

The biochemical reactions of smooth muscle cells that occur in atherosclerosis will be discussed in chapter 6.

Macrophages

Macrophages are present in normal intima at a low frequency. They may increase in number in adaptive intimal thickening and in atherosclerotic lesions. The function of these cells in normal intima is uncertain but could include the following.

1. Remodelling of the intima.

   Macrophages can synthesise and secrete the metaloproteases, collagenase and elastase and hence can modify extra cellular matrix. Synthesis and secretion of growth factors by macrophages for endothelial cells and smooth muscle cells could increase turnover of these cells.

2. Inflammatory response and scavenger function.

   Macrophages are responsible for the phagocytosis and cytolysis of bacteria and tumour cells in infected tissue. In the arterial intima macrophages are responsible for the phagocytosis and removal of dead cells and immune complexes, removal of plasma proteins and lipoproteins.

   Macrophages secrete cytokines that attract lymphocytes to sites of injury. Thus, macrophages in atherosclerotic lesions may be responsible for the influx of T- cells which are seen in more advanced lesions.

3. Immune response.

   Binding and presentation of antigens, cytokine and growth factor production related to the immune response.

The biochemical reactions occurring in macrophages during atherosclerosis will be discussed in chapter 6.

Extracellular matrix

The extracellular matrix components have a number of important physiological functions. These include:

1. Arterial permeability: the transfer of essential nutrients across the intima.

   Essential nutrients from the blood can pass across the intima to the cells within the intima and to the underlying media. All plasma proteins are present in the intima at concentrations dependent upon the protein's molecular weight and concentration in the blood. Thus it is perfectly normal for LDL to be found in the intima but if the concentration of this lipoprotein is elevated in the blood, its concentration in the intima will also be increased.

   The proteoglycans of the extracellular matrix act in part as a filtering mechanism and also as an ion exchange system because of the negatively charged sulphate and carboxyl groups on the glycosaminoglycan chains. LDL binds with a high affinity to chondroitin sulphate proteoglycan. The interaction between the lipoprotein and the extracellular matrix proteoglycan may be responsible for retarding the transfer of the lipoprotein across the intima: the retention of lipoprotein in the intima will be discussed further in chapter 6.

2. Structural integrity of the intima.

   The chondroitin sulphate proteoglycan and hyaluronate network provides the intima with its strength and compression properties. The collagen and elastin fibres provide further structural strengthening. Cells within the intima are held in the extracellular matrix by cell associated heparin sulphate proteoglycan.

3. Regulation of cell proliferation.

   Increased synthesis of proteoglycans and also collagen and thrombospondin accompanies the proliferation of smooth muscle cells. However heparin sulphate proteoglycan inhibits cell proliferation. This proteoglycan may bind and influence the activity of growth factors and hence help to regulate cell proliferation.

2.4 Atherosclerotic lesions

Lesion initiation

Various factors are known to predispose the development of atherosclerosis with clinical symptoms (these factors are discussed in chapter 3). However, while considerable progress has been made in elucidating the mechanisms of lesion initiation and progression some aspects are still not fully understood.

Elevated plasma lipoprotein concentrations have been shown to be associated with increased concentrations in the intima and may stimulate certain cell reactions that cause some of the changes that are observed in atherosclerotic lesion formation. Regions where lipoprotein concentrations in the intima are high may be those exposed to mechanical forces which favour increased residence time of circulating lipoproteins and cells at the endothelial surface. These regions, frequently located at certain arterial branch points, are referred to as **lesion-prone sites** since these are sites where more advanced lesions are frequently found. The position and nature of these sites suggest that haemodynamic forces have a role in facilitating lesion formation. Lipoproteins within the intima may undergo chemical modification that facilitates their uptake by macrophages. Normally the artery wall contains few macrophages, but in diseased tissue, macrophages accumulate: these derive from circulating monocytes which first adhere to the endothelial cells and then penetrate into the subendothelial space. Monocyte adhesion and transmigration to the intima, lipoprotein modification within the intima, and the interaction between different cells within atherosclerotic lesions will be discussed in chapter 6.

Types of atherosclerotic lesions

A classification of human atherosclerotic lesions has been made on the basis of specific morphological characteristics. From observations of the structure of the atherosclerotic artery it is thought that types I, II and III lesions may be successive stages in the development of atherosclerosis and that type III is the bridge between type II and advanced lesions which may give rise to clinical symptoms. Each of these three types of lesion is focal and contains an abnormal accumulation of lipid, mainly in the form of cholesterol ester. Advanced atherosclerotic lesions are divided histologically into types IV, V and VI; in these lesions the accumulation of lipid, cells and matrix is accompanied by structural disorganisation, repair and thickening of the intima and deformity of the artery wall. Quantitative data on lesion prevalence in humans has been obtained mainly from autopsy of accident victims.

Diagrams of the types of atherosclerotic lesions are shown in figure 2.4.

Type I

Type I lesions are most frequent in infants and children but may also be found in adults. These lesions comprise isolated groups of macrophages containing many lipid droplets, in the intima: these are known as **macrophage foam cells** (see figure 2.5).

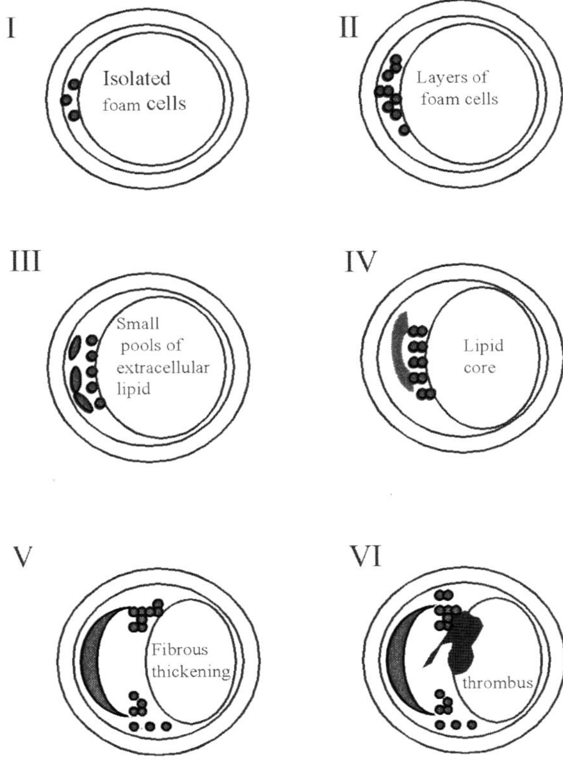

Figure 2.4
Different types of atherosclerotic lesion. (Adapted from H.C.Stary *et al.*, 1994)

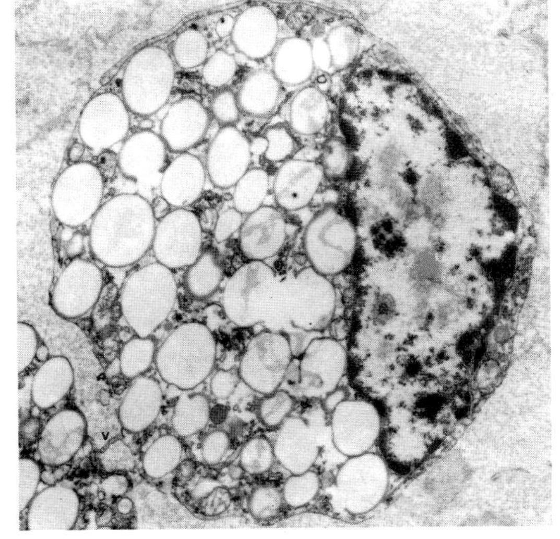

Figure 2.5
A macrophage foam cell. Electron micrograph (x 12600)

In a survey of 69 children who died before the age of 5 years macrophages were observed in the intima of the coronary artery examined in 94% of the children. In the first 8 months of life, 45% of infants had macrophage foam cells in the coronary arteries and macrophages without lipid droplets were increased two fold. However the percentage of children with macrophage foam cells decreased in those above 8 months old (17%). It was pointed out that there was no evidence to conclude that those infants with intimal foam cells would necessarily have developed fatty streaks or atheroma in those regions of the artery wall had they survived.

The observation that the earliest changes in the artery wall in hypercholesterolemic animals is the appearance of intimal macrophage foam cells, suggests that the early development of the disease is similar in humans and experimental animals.

Type II

These consist mainly of layers of macrophage foam cells, rather than isolated groups of these lipid filled cells. Intimal smooth muscle cells also contain lipid droplets. A greater number of macrophages without lipid droplets may be present than in type I lesions. Some T lymphocytes and mast cells may also be present.

Most of the lipid of type II lesions is intracellular, mainly in macrophages. Some extracellular lipid droplets may be visible. The major lipid present in type II lesions is cholesterol ester with oleate (35%) and linoleate (26%) being the main fatty acid, esterified to cholesterol.

Some type II lesions are grossly visible in post-mortem arteries as fatty, yellow coloured streaks. These **fatty streaks** stain red with certain dyes such as Sudan IV or oil-red O. Similar lesions can be induced experimentally in animals.

Type II lesions can be divided into type IIa, which occur in lesion prone (progression prone) regions, and IIb, which do not progress, progress slowly or progress only in persons with elevated plasma lipoproteins. Morphologically these subgroups differ; type IIa have more smooth muscle cells, more extracellular matrix of collocated intimal thickening, greater accumulation of lipoprotein and macrophages and deep intimal location of foam cells and extracellular lipid droplets. If foam cells are found mainly in the lower region of a thickened intima these lesions may not be so readily visible with *en-face* histological techniques.

In post mortem aorta of children aged 2-15 years, 99% had type II lesions. The extent of type II lesions increased in the descending aorta up to the age of 20 years. In the abdominal aorta the extent of these lesions increased up to the age of 30 years, when it exceeded the extent in the thoracic artery. The locations in the aorta in which type II lesions develop into advanced lesions is on the left and right posterolateral walls between the orifice of the inferior mesenteric artery and the bifurcation of the common iliac arteries.

Type II lesions are seen around puberty in the coronary arteries. In a study of young people, 65% of those aged 12-14 years had type I or II lesions and 8% had more advanced lesions in the left proximal coronary artery. Advanced lesions tend to occur first in the intima of the left anterior coronary artery that is opposite the flow divider of the main bifurcation.

Type III

In addition to the morphological features of type II lesions there are multiple separate extracellular lipid pools that lie below the layers of macrophages and macrophage foam cells and disrupt the coherence of structural smooth muscle cells in the intima. The lipid in these lesions contains more free cholesterol, fatty acid, sphingomyelin, lysophosphatidylcholine and triacylglycerol than type II lesions. The change in lipid composition probably reflects the increasing amount of extracellular lipid.

Type IV

This is also known as an **atheroma** and comprises the features of type III lesion with a dense accumulation of extracellular lipid termed the lipid core; this may contain cholesterol crystals and calcium deposits. Between the lipid core and the endothelial surface, the intima contains macrophages and smooth muscle cells with and without lipid droplets. Capillaries may border the lipid core and often macrophages, smooth muscle cells and lymphocytes are more densely accumulated at the lesion periphery.

The lipid core may result from the accumulation of the remains of many dead foam cells. In man, type IV lesions are frequently seen after about the age of thirty. In medium sized arteries these lesions do not significantly impede blood flow and are thus clinically silent. If, however, the lesion develops fissures thrombosis may ensue and clinical symptoms may arise.

Type V

These lesions have prominent new fibrous connective tissue. New tissue, which may comprises increased collagen and smooth muscle cells rich in rough endoplasmic reticulum, may be laid down in an attempt to repair the damage to the intimal organisation produced by the lipid core, or the incorporation of a thrombus remnant into the lesion. Capillaries at the margin of the lipid core may be larger than in type IV lesions and they may be present in the new connective tissue. Type V lesions can be sub-divided: types Va are atherosclerotic lesions with the morphology just described. These lesions may be multi-layered with several lipid cores separated by layers of fibrous connective tissue. If the lipid core and other parts of the lesion are calcified these are type Vb. If the lipid core is absent and lipid deposits minimal these are type Vc. Type V lesions may be associated with an accompanying disruption of the adjacent media.

Type VI

These are type IV or V lesions that have been modified by either, disruption of the surface (type VIa), haematoma or haemorrhage (type VIb) or thrombosis (type VIc).

Disruption of the lesion surface, by fissures or tears of the surface or ulceration involving loss of endothelial cells may vary in severity and may lead to hemorrhage or thrombi formation. The latter may be the cause of the occlusion of a vessel or it may be incorporated into the structure of the lesion leading to further narrowing of the artery lumen.

Atherosclerotic aneurysm

Distinct localised outward bulges or **aneurysms** are associated with type VI lesions in which the intima is eroded, the extracellular intimal matrix is altered and media may also be modified. These aneurysms may rupture with fatal consequences.

Coronary thrombosis

Thrombosis, occurring above an atherosclerotic lesion, is frequently the cause of acute coronary occlusion, sudden death, unstable angina and acute coronary insufficiency. In 1974-1979 a prospective clinical study was carried out in which radioactive fibrinogen was administered to patients admitted to a coronary care unit. In the fatal cases, autoradiagraphy showed the distribution of fibrin in thrombotic material formed after the introduction of isotopically labelled fibrinogen (figure 2.6) It was found that 56 out of 57 cases had thrombotic occlusion of the coronary arteries. Administration of thrombolytic drugs is now a routine part of the treatment of patients in coronary care units.

Development and progression of atherosclerosis

There is a progressive impairment of endothelial function as atherosclerosis progresses. While endothelial dysfunction may well be

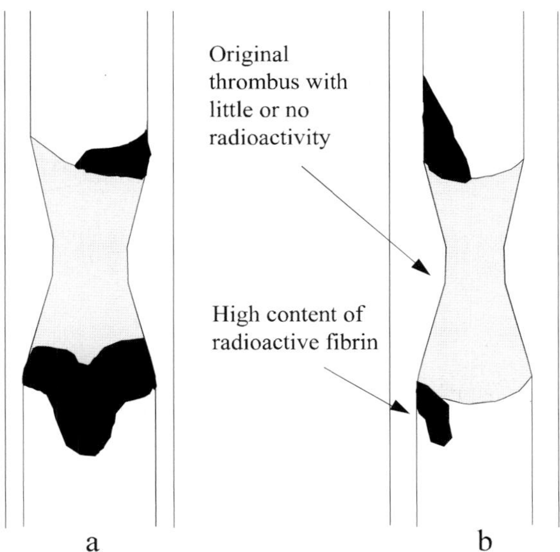

Figure 2.6 Acute coronary occlusion: distribution of ^{125}I-labelled fibrin in post-mortem sample. (Adapted from W.F.M.Fulten, 1993)

an early occurrence in atherosclerosis the appearance of gross physical damage to the endothelium is a later process. The coronary arteries of six human hearts, removed from patients with severe atherosclerosis undergoing heart transplant, were examined, after perfusion with glutaraldehyde, by scanning electron microscopy. This showed that there was no damage to the endothelium over fatty streaks, although the surface was raised through accumulation of lipid. However endothelial denudation did occur over more advanced lesions. Platelets were seen on the surface where the endothelium was damaged. All patients had morphologically intact endothelium in regions where lesions were absent.

In puberty the frequency of occurrence of early atherosclerotic lesions declines and the number of more advanced lesions increases (see figure 2.7). This observation suggests the progression of the early lesions to the more advanced types. The ultrastructure of the various types of lesions supports this hypothesis.

2.6 Conclusion

Some insight into the early events of atherosclerosis, i.e. the process of initiation of atheromatous lesions has been obtained by studying atherosclerosis development in animal models and from studies of aortic cells in culture and co-culture. These early events probably represent what occurs in the human artery *in vivo*. From such studies it is known what conditions predispose to atherogenesis and under what conditions lesion development occurs. The continued exposure to these conditions

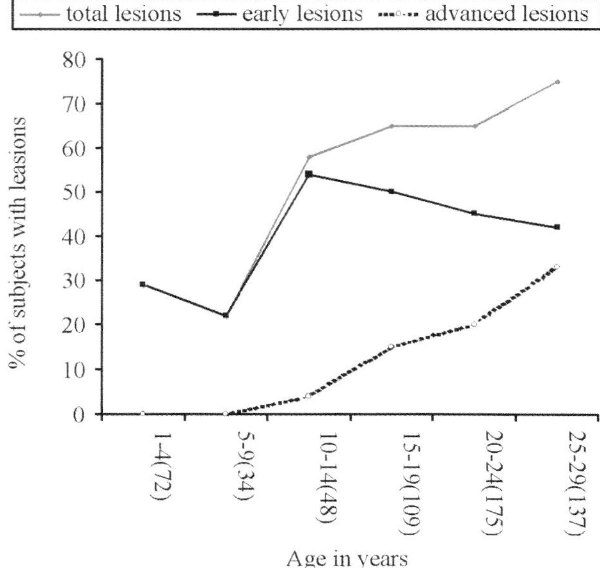

Figure 2.7 Frequency of occurrence of different types of atherosclerotic lesions in coronary arteries. Adapted from H.C.Stary, 1989)

Lesions in the left coronary artery of humans who died between full term birth and age 29 years (total =565). Number of subjects in each age group is shown in parentheses. Mean interval between death and fixation with glutaraldehyde was 9.5 hours. Details of eccentric thickening and atherosclerotic lesions obtained from sequential cross sections, examined by light and electron microscopy.

may lead to progression of lesions to the more advanced forms which will lead to ischemia of tissues supplied by the atherosclerotic vessels and clinical symptoms of atherosclerotic disease. From studies in man and from animal studies, there is evidence that under certain circumstances atherosclerotic lesions reduce in size, usually with gradual disappearance of lipid; this process of regression will be discussed further in chapter 11.

As lesion initiation may occur in childhood and development, progression and regression of atherosclerotic lesions may occur very slowly, preventative measures should be taken during childhood or early adulthood to avoid clinical illness in later years and to prevent premature fatalities from atherosclerotic disease.

Key references

Methods of investigation of atherosclerosis

Merickel, M.B. *et al.* (1993) Non-invasive quantitative evaluation of atherosclerosis using MRI and image analysis. Arterioscler.Thromb. 13, 1180-1186

Suckling, K.E. & Jackson, B. (1993) Animal models of human lipid metabolism. Progress in Lipid Research, 32, 1-24

Nistor, A., Bull, A., Filip, D.A. and Radu A.(1987) The hyperlipidemic hamster as a model of experimental atherosclerosis. Atherosclerosis 68, 159-173

Rubin, E.M. and Smith, D.J. (1994) Atherosclerosis in mice: getting to the heart of a polygenic disorder. Trends in Genetics 10, 199-203

Proteoglycans of the extracellular matrix

Hurt-Camejo, E. *et al.* (1997) Cellular consequences of the association of apoB lipoproteins with proteoglycans. Potential contribution to atherogenesis. Arterioslerosis, Thrombosis and Vascular Biolology. 17, 1011-1017

Types of atherosclerotic lesions and atherosclerotic lesion pathology

Stary, H.C. *et al.* (1994) A definition of initial, fatty streak and intermediate lesions of atherosclerosis. Arteriosclerosis and Thrombosis. 14, 840-856

Stary, H.C. *et al.* (1995) A definition of advanced types of atherosclerotic lesions and a histological classification of atherosclerosis. Arterioslerosis, Thrombosis and Vascular Biolology. 15, 1512-1531

Morphology of the endothelium over atherosclerotic plaques in human coronary arteries. (1988) M.J.Davies, N.Woolf, P.M.Rowles and J.Pepper. British Heart Journal. 60, 459-464

Ball, R.Y. *et al.* (1995) Evidence that death of macrophage foam cells contribute to the lipid core of atheroma. Atherosclerosis 114, 45-54

Ross, R. (1993) The pathogenesis of atherosclerosis: a perspective for the 1990s. Nature 362, 801-809

Lesion prevalence in humans

Stary, H.C. (1987) Macrophages, macrophage foam cells and eccentric intimal thickening in the coronary arteries of younger children. Atherosclerosis 64, 91-108

Stary, H.C. (1989) Evolution and progression of atherosclerotic lesions in coronary arteries in children and young adults. Arteriosclerosis. 9 suppl 1, 19-32

Coronary thrombosis

Fulten, W.F.M. (1993) Pathological concepts in acute coronary thrombosis: relevance to treatment. British Heart Journal. 73, 403-408

3 Risk Factors

3.1 Introduction

There is no single cause of atherosclerosis; it is a multi-factorial disease with a wide range of **risk factors** associated with it. Explaining the concept of risk factors represents one of the most difficult tasks in health education. All to frequently people will know of individuals who, despite the presence of supposed risk factors, have lived long and healthy lives. A risk factor is exactly what it says; a factor that increases the likelihood, or risk, of developing a disease, or, in the case of atherosclerosis, increases the rate at which the disease develops.

In this chapter we will look briefly at some of the methods used to identify risk factors for disease in general and will then go through the evidence that specific factors are associated with the development of cardiovascular disease. By necessity we can only give a brief overview of epidemiological techniques and the reader is directed elsewhere for more, fuller accounts.

3.2 Epidemiological methods

Epidemiology is the study of the occurrence of disease within populations. A wide range of techniques is used to gather such information depending on the specific hypothesis to be tested and the frequency of the disease outcome in the population. However in the real world, other factors such as cost and length of time available in which to perform the study, unfortunately, very often become the first consideration. In general epidemiological studies can be divided into Descriptive (or Ecological) Studies, Analytical Studies and Experimental Studies. Each of these is briefly described below.

Descriptive studies

A descriptive study will normally describe the distribution of a disease within or between, populations and relate this to the occurrence or distribution of putative risk factors. Such a study will rely on data, which is already available and consequently can often be performed on large numbers of subjects. The occurrence of a disease is often considered based on geographical location, ethnic group, occupational or social class groups or over specific time periods. One particularly valuable form of Ecological Study is that of Migrants, where people of similar genetic background can be compared in different environments. The advantage of descriptive studies is that they can involve large numbers of people relatively cheaply. The major disadvantages are that the researcher often has little insight into the quality of data and such studies may give no indication of possible cause and effect.

Analytical studies

Analytical Studies, which often arise from the results of a Descriptive Study, are designed to test a specific hypothesis, i.e. can a definite association be made between a possible risk factor and a disease. It is important to note that epidemiology will not reveal the cause of a disease only reveals associations. One vital part of interpreting epidemiological data is the identification of confounding variables, something, which may indirectly link the risk factor to the disease. In general the most persuasive epidemiological data is that which indicates the correct direction of the association. The best design for such a study is that of a **Cohort Study**. A group of people, free from the disease state being studied, are chosen to be representative of a specified population. They are then screened for the risk factor (s) to be tested and, after a predefined time period, they are re-evaluated for the occurrence of the disease in question. The occurrence of the potential risk factors, at the initial screening, in those who developed the disease is compared to the occurrence *in* those who did not develop the disease. The disadvantage of Cohort Studies is that they tend to be expensive to perform, as they may have to run over many years. In the case of particularly rare diseases such studies may not be possible because of the number of subjects and the length of time required to obtain sufficient numbers in the "disease group". These diseases are usually best studied in **Case Control Studies**. In the latter, people known to have the disease in question are compared to matched, disease-free, controls. Patients with the disease can be found in hospitals or clinics and compared with matched controls, who may be family members or friends from the same environment. The big disadvantage of case control studies is that a cause and effect relationship cannot be directly demonstrated.

Experimental studies

The most direct evidence that a risk factor is directly associated with the development of a disease is an Experimental or **Intervention Study**. Here exposure to the risk factor is either increased or decreased and the outcome, in terms of development of the disease is observed. The major limitation of such studies is an ethical one. One cannot undertake an intervention that is likely to increase the expectation that the treated individuals will develop a serious disease. Furthermore, even in experiments where the intervention may protect the individuals, it may be unethical to leave the control group untreated.

Table 3.1 Advantages and disadvantages of different sorts of epidemiological studies

Type of study	*Advantages*	*Disadvantages*
Descriptive	Can study large numbers of subjects. Relatively inexpensive.	Often no control over quality of data. No indication of a cause: effect relationship.
Cohort	Strong evidence for a cause: effect relationship may be obtained.	Expensive and may have to be performed over a prolonged time period. Not appropriate for rare diseases.
Case Control	Can be used to study rare disease. Relatively inexpensive.	No indication of cause: effect relationship.
Experimental	Can directly indicate the relationship between a single variable and disease occurrence.	Design must decrease disease incidence. May be unethical to fail to treat the control group. Expensive.

3.3 Epidemiological studies of risk factors for CHD

There have been numerous studies looking at the relationship of potential risk factors to the development of atherosclerotic disease. Obviously not all of them can be mentioned here. Instead four major studies which have been important in defining potential risk factors will be discussed.

The Framingham Study

An epidemiological study which has made probably the most significant contribution to the understanding of atherosclerotic disease was that carried out in the town of Framingham in USA. This has become known as the **Framingham Study**. This Cohort Study, beginning in 1950, studied over 5,000 men and women for a period of 24 years. The effect of various potential risk factors on the development of the major clinical manifestations of atherosclerosis, namely, coronary heart disease, stroke or peripheral arterial disease, was determined. Clinical evaluation of subjects was carried out by skilled physicians, and diagnosis made from interviews with the subjects and from data from some non-invasive measurements, such as electrocardiograms. Subjects were seen every

2 years, for as long as they were living, for the 24 years of the study. Various hypotheses were proposed at the outset of the study and some of these are listed in table 3.2. Some other hypotheses were later proposed and tested using the data collected. The results obtained for factors which were found to be associated with the development of atherosclerotic disease will be discussed below.

Table 3.2 Hypothesis and results of the Framingham Study

Hypothesis proposed for investigation in the Framingham Study	*Hypothesis supported?*
1. Coronary heart disease increases with **age** (as do other manifestations of atherosclerotic disease). It occurs earlier and more frequently in the male sex.	Yes
2. Persons with **hypertension** develop coronary heart disease at a greater rate than those who are normotensive	Yes
3. Elevated **blood cholesterol level** is associated with an increased risk of coronary heart disease.	Yes, in men and in older women
4. Tobacco **smoking** is associated with an increased occurrence of coronary heart disease.	Yes, in men
5. Habitual use of **alcohol** is associated with increased incidence of coronary heart disease.	No
6. Increased **physical activity** is associated with a decrease in the development of coronary heart disease.	No, however data suggested that a sedentary life was to be avoided.
7. An increase in **body weight** predisposes to coronary heart disease.	Yes
8. There is an increased rate of development of coronary heart disease in patients with **diabetes** mellitus	Yes

1. Effect of age and sex on incidence of atherosclerotic disease

In the Framingham Study the incidence of coronary heart disease, myocardial infarct and angina pectoris increased with increasing age in both men and women. The incidence in men was significantly higher than in women for each age group considered (4-5 year intervals between

30 and 59 years). The incidence of cerebral vascular disease increased with age but the differences between male and female were not so marked as for coronary heart disease and were absent in the upper age groups (50-54 and 55-59 years.). The incidence of peripheral artery disease, as measured by intermittent claudication, was similar in pattern to that of coronary artery disease, i.e. increasing with age but higher in men than women for each age group considered.

The presence of one form of atherosclerotic disease increased the likelihood of the patient suffering from another form of the disease. For example, patients who had had a stroke were four times as likely to suffer from myocardial infarct as those who had not had a stroke. As angina pectoris and myocardial infarct are expressions of the same underlying pathology it is not surprising that the incidence of myocardial infarcts was found to be six times higher in people who had suffered from angina than in the normal population.

2. Hypertension and atherosclerotic disease

The measurement of blood pressure is complicated by variability in a single subject. Therefore in the Framingham Study at each biennial examination a subject's blood pressure was taken initially by a nurse, then by the physician at the beginning and the end of the physical examination. The blood pressure was recorded as normotensive if both pressures recorded by the physician were less than 140/90mmHg, hypertensive if both pressures recorded by the physicians were 160/95mmHg or above and borderline if the values fell between. The results showed, in both men and women, that the incidence of coronary heart disease progressively increased from those with normal blood pressure, to those with borderline hypertension, to those classed as hypertensive. A similar pattern of incidence was seen for both myocardial infarct and angina pectoris. The annual incidence of coronary heart disease related to these blood pressure categories is shown in figure 3.1.

3. Blood cholesterol concentrations and atherosclerotic disease

High concentrations of cholesterol in atheromatous lesions in human aortas and the association of familial hypercholesterolaemia with cardiovascular disease (see chapter 5) provided support for the hypothesis that blood cholesterol plays an important role in the development of atherosclerosis. This hypothesis was supported further by data collected in the Framingham Study and corroborated by other epidemiological studies.

Observations made in the Framingham Study showed a strong association of serum cholesterol with the incidence of coronary heart disease. Serum cholesterol showed a normal distribution in men that

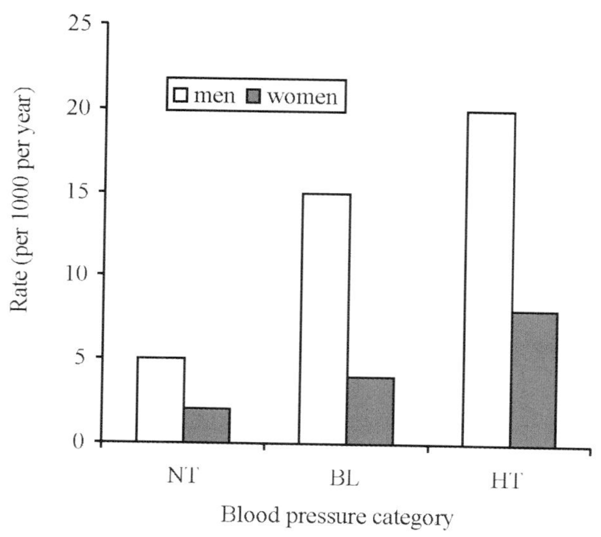

Figure 3.1
Effect of blood pressure category on the incidence of coronary heart disease. Data from the Framingham Study. NT, normotensive; BL, borderline; HT, hypertensive

was little affected by age in the age span studied (30-59yr). While a normal distribution for serum cholesterol was obtained in women, the mean value varied with age. Serum cholesterol was lower in women than men in the 30-39 yr. age group but higher than men in the 50-59 yr. age group. In men the incidence of coronary heart disease increased with increasing serum cholesterol and with age (figure 3.2).

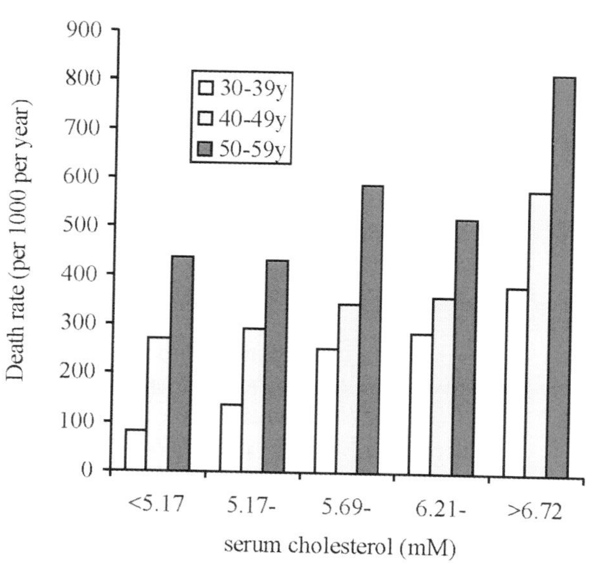

Figure 3.2
Effect of serum cholesterol on the incidence of coronary heart disease. Data from 24 year follow-up in Framingham Study

In men of 30-39 yr., with a serum cholesterol greater than 6.7mM, the relative risk of developing coronary heart disease was four times the risk seen in those with a serum cholesterol below 5.2mM. In women, there was a correlation between the serum cholesterol and the incidence of coronary heart disease in the 40-49 yr. age group. The incidence was low in the 30-39 yr. age group and apparently unrelated to serum cholesterol. In the 50-59 yr. age group the incidence of coronary heart disease was much higher but again appeared to be unrelated to serum cholesterol.

There was a similarity in the patterns of incidence of total coronary heart disease, myocardial infarct and angina pectoris with cholesterol levels. The relationship of serum cholesterol to the incidence of cerebral infarct was equivocal. It was not possible from this data to conclude that the incidence of thrombolytic stroke was related to serum cholesterol. However elevated serum cholesterol did appear to play a role in the development of peripheral arterial disease.

In men the average cholesterol concentration did not change with age. In a particular age group the incidence of coronary heart disease was proportional to the serum cholesterol. In other words serum cholesterol was confirmed as an independent risk factor. This also applied to women in the 40-49yr. age group in the Framingham Study. As discussed in section 3.3 below, it is now known that the distribution of cholesterol between different plasma lipoproteins is at least as important as total plasma cholesterol.

4. Effect of smoking on atherosclerotic disease

A strong relationship between cigarette smoking and the incidence of coronary heart disease was seen in men although the effect was less in older subjects. Thus, in young males the incidence of coronary heart disease in smokers was twice that of non-smokers. In women no significant effect of smoking was observed. If smoking habits, in men, were assessed nearer to the time of coronary heart disease diagnosis, the rate in smokers was three fold that of non-smokers in the 30-39 yr. and 40-49 yr. age groups and two-fold in the 50-59yr. age group.

When differences in smoking habits was taken into account it was found that the rate of sudden death in smokers was twice that of non-smokers in all age groups. This relationship was not lost with age. In smokers, in the younger age groups, the risk of developing angina pectoris was two-fold greater than in non-smokers but this was less evident in older subjects. There was a higher rate of cerebral vascular accidents in smokers but the differences were not statistically significant. The incidence of intermittent claudication in male smokers was two-three fold that seen in non-smokers. A two-fold increase in incidence of intermittent claudication in older women was revealed when the smoking habits were assessed at a time near to the diagnosis of atherosclerotic disease.

5. Obesity and atherosclerotic disease

The body weight is a function of height, body build, sex, degree of muscular development and degree of adiposity. In the Framingham Study a relative weight was calculated. The weight of each individual was compared to the median weight of all persons examined in the same age, sex and height category. For example a subject with a relative weight of 130 was 30% above the median weight of his or her age, sex and height group. A subject with a relative weight of 80 was 20% below the median weight. This method, while valuable within a population, is not useful for comparison of different populations who may have different nutritional status.

Male subjects, who were 20% or more above the median weight, were about two-fold more at risk of developing coronary heart disease than those below the median weight. Those below 80% relative weight were at a lower risk than those of median weight. In women, a similar relationship of weight to incidence was observed. In both sexes, the incidence rate of angina pectoris was significantly higher the greater the relative weight and the age of onset of symptoms was lower the greater the relative weight. For myocardial infarct there was no relationship between relative weight and incidence in the 30-39yr. age group but in older men and women the incidence was significantly higher in the overweight group than the median weight group. The risk of sudden death increased in overweight men. In women the incidence of sudden death was low and evaluation of the effect of weight on risk could not be made. The incidence rate for cerebral vascular accidents was greater the higher the relative weight. The incidence rate in subjects 20% or more above the median weight was two to three fold that of subjects below the median weight. There was no evidence that intermittent claudication increased with increasing weight. In each age decade, for both men and women, body weight was related to blood pressure. Both systolic and diastolic blood pressure increased significantly with increasing weight.

6. Diabetes and atherosclerotic disease

Based on the diagnosis at the initial examination the subsequent incidence of coronary heart disease over 24 years was significantly higher in diabetics than in non -diabetics. In men, the incidence rate for coronary heart disease in diabetics was two-fold higher than in non-diabetics, while in women it was five-fold. The rate of myocardial infarcts was two-fold higher in male diabetics and six-fold higher in female diabetics compared to their non-diabetic counterparts. There was a greater risk of sudden death or stroke in diabetics than in non-diabetics. The average annual incidence of intermittent claudicication was five-fold higher in men and up to nine-fold higher in women, with diabetes. Thus diabetes is an important risk factor for the development of atherosclerotic disease.

Low density and high density lipoproteins

Numerous epidemiological studies, including the Framingham Study described above, have shown a strong positive correlation of serum cholesterol and the incidence of coronary heart disease within particular populations. Other studies, such as the Seven Countries Study, showed this to be true when international comparisons were made.

As will be discussed in chapter 4, cholesterol is carried in the blood in particles called lipoproteins. The major cholesterol carrying lipoproteins are low-density lipoprotein (LDL) and high-density lipoprotein (HDL). Since the 1950s, when the newly invented ultracentrifuge was used to separate the plasma lipoproteins, it has been suggested that these two types of lipoproteins have different relationships to coronary heart disease. In an appraisal of several epidemiological studies and from data from their own study, the Framingham Study, Kannel and co-workers proposed that LDL cholesterol was a better predictor of the risk of coronary heart disease than total serum cholesterol.

In contrast, an inverse association of HDL cholesterol with the incidence of coronary heart disease has been found. It was not until the 1970s that the association of HDL with atherosclerosis was firmly established. Before then the relatively costly and time consuming ultracentrifugation techniques meant that most studies were small and lacking in statistical power. However, the discovery of a quick and inexpensive precipitation technique to isolate HDL meant that large studies could easily be performed. Such techniques were introduced into the Framingham Study as well as several other large epidemiological studies. In the British Regional Heart Study, it was found that, if the population was divided into quintiles (fifths) based on their HDL cholesterol concentration, those in the lowest quintile had a two-fold increase of risk of ischaemic heart disease compared with those in the highest. It was estimated that for every 0.026mM increase in HDL cholesterol there was a 2.5% reduction in risk of ischaemic heart disease. In a study of older men and women in Framingham, in whom total cholesterol was not a particularly good indicator of risk, HDL cholesterol was found to exhibit a strong negative association with the incidence of coronary heart disease. Thus, HDL cholesterol concentration is an independent risk factor that is inversely related to the risk of coronary heart disease.

Further discussion of the association of lipoprotein sub-fractions and apolipoproteins with the occurrence and extent of coronary heart disease will be deferred until the metabolism of lipoproteins has been discussed.

3.4 Intervention studies

If having a high level of total, or LDL, cholesterol is a risk factor for cardiovascular disease then does reducing your cholesterol reduce your risk? While the obvious answer would seem to be yes, this has actually taken a long time to prove. A number of large intervention studies in the 1970s produced inconclusive results. One such study is described below. It is only recently, with the development of highly potent cholesterol-lowering drugs, that the question has finally been resolved.

The Multiple Risk Factor Intervention Trial (MRFIT)

In the early 1970's 356,000 American men were screened for an intervention study. Those men found to be at the greatest risk, in terms of high serum cholesterol, high blood pressure and smokers were recruited on to the trial (12,866 men aged 35-57 years). They were randomly assigned to two groups, the intervention group and the control group. The former were counselled and treated to reduce blood pressure, advised to reduce cigarette smoking and given dietary advice to lower cholesterol while the latter had only the usual health care. During the six years of the study, there were significant reductions in each of the risk factors in each group. However, the magnitude of these changes was consistently greater in the intervention group than the controls. At the end of the study mortality from coronary heart disease was observed to be non-significantly lower in the intervention group than the controls (17.9/1,000 *vs* 19.3/1,000, respectively). In addition, a non-significant rise in "non-coronary heart disease" deaths was seen in the intervention group, such that overall mortality was no different between the two groups. The results of this massive (both in terms of numbers and of expense) trial led many to question the efficacy of risk factor reduction in prevention of coronary heart disease.

However, the MRFIT was important because results obtained at the initial screening and deaths occurring in the following six years provided further evidence for the relationship of serum cholesterol and the incidence of coronary heart disease. The death rate was directly proportional to the serum cholesterol levels observed at the initial screening i.e. the risk of developing fatal coronary heart disease increased as the serum cholesterol increased. It was calculated from the data that a 1% increase in serum cholesterol could increase the risk of death from coronary heart disease by 2%.

This trial also showed the relationship between several risk factors. As was observed in the Framingham Study the increase of coronary heart deaths with increasing cholesterol was further increased with age. Figure 3.3 shows the relationship of coronary heart deaths with cholesterol in

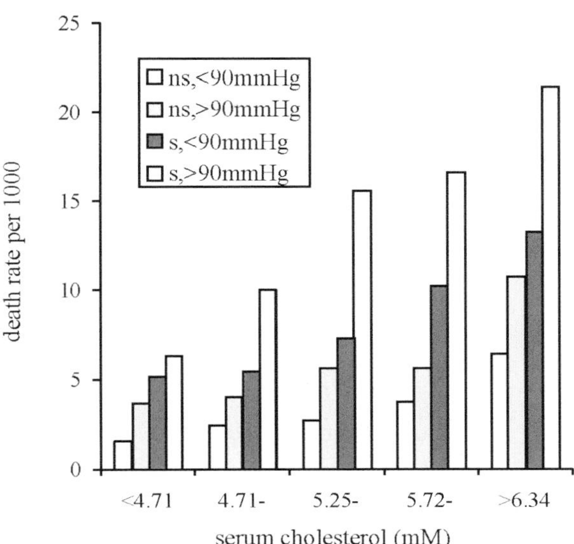

Figure 3.3 Effect of serum cholesterol, blood pressure and smoking on coronary heart disease. Data from the Multiple Risk Factor Intervention Trial (MRFIT). ns, non-smokers; s, smokers. Figures are for diastolic blood pressure

non smokers and smokers and in those with diastolic blood pressure below 90mmHg and those with diastolic blood pressure above this value. Thus, the risk of developing fatal coronary heart disease increased as the serum cholesterol increased and the risk was greater in smokers or those persons with elevated blood pressure. Those most at risk smoked, had elevated blood pressure and serum cholesterol concentrations.

The Scandinavian Simvastatin Survival Study (4S)

The equivocal results of the MRFIT and other intervention trials of the 1970s and 1980s led some researchers and clinicians to doubt the benefit of reducing plasma cholesterol. However by the 1990s a new, powerful tool for cholesterol lowering became widely available. A new class of drugs, the HMGCoA reductase inhibitors, was shown to produce large sustainable decreases in total and LDL cholesterol with very few side effects reported. In 1994 the results of the Scandinavian Simvastatin Survival Study (4S) gave one of the clearest indications of the benefits of cholesterol reduction. This was a secondary intervention trial, meaning that the subjects involved had already suffered a coronary event, and the aim was to investigate the effect of cholesterol lowering on the occurrence of further such events. 4,444 patients took part in the trial, they were divided into a placebo group, and a group treated with the drug, Simvastatin. Patients were followed for a median of 5.4 years and the treated group achieved and maintained a 35% reduction in LDL cholesterol. This was associated with a 30% decrease in total mortality compared to the control group, predominantly due to a fall in deaths from coronary heart disease. Equally important was the fact that there was no indication of an increase in deaths from other causes.

The West of Scotland Study

The results of the 4S secondary prevention trial were closely followed by those of a primary prevention trial, the West of Scotland Study. This was an experimental, double blind study, designed to determine if a reduction of cholesterol, by administration of another HMGCoA reductase inhibitor, Pravastatin, reduced the incidence of coronary heart disease. The study involved 6,595 men aged 45-64 years with a mean plasma cholesterol of 7.0 $\pm$0.6mM (272 $\pm$23 mg/dl), but without history of previous myocardial infarction, who received 40mg Pravastatin per day or placebo. Pravastatin was found to lower plasma cholesterol by 20% and LDL cholesterol by 26%. No change was observed with placebo. There were 248 coronary events i.e. non-fatal myocardial infarcts and deaths from coronary heart disease, in the placebo group and 174 in the group taking Pravastatin (a relative reduction of 31%, 95% confidence limit). Similar reductions were seen in the number of non-fatal myocardial infarcts and in deaths from all cardiovascular disease. There was no increase in deaths from non-cardiovascular disease causes in the Pravastatin group. In fact, there was a 22% reduction in the risk of death, from any cause, in this group. Thus in hypercholesterolaemic men a reduction in cholesterol was significantly associated with a reduction in the risk of coronary heart disease.

3.5 Conclusion

A word of caution: a person with high serum cholesterol is not necessarily going to suffer a heart attack or die of stroke. However he, or she, is at a higher risk of doing so than a person with a lower cholesterol level. Other factors in the lifestyle of that person have to be taken into account in establishing the overall risk of developing symptoms of atherosclerotic disease. Chapter 11 gives examples of countries where plasma cholesterol concentrations are not particularly different but the incidence of coronary heart disease varies substantially. Thus, other factors appear to protect some populations against developing coronary heart disease even in the presence of moderately high serum cholesterol levels. These differences in mortality may be related to significant differences in diet of different countries, which will be considered in more detail in later chapters.

Key references

Epidemiology

Friedman, Gary D. (1994) Primer of Epidemiology. McGraw-Hill, Inc.

The Framingham Study

Dawber, T.R. (1980)The Framingham Study. The epidemiology of atherosclerotic disease. Havard University Press

Low Density and High Density Lipoprotein

Simons, L.A. (1986) Interrelationships of lipids and lipoproteins with coronary artery disease mortality in 19 countries. American Journal of Cardiology 57, 5G-10G

Kannel, W.B., Castelli, W.P. and Gordon, T. (1979) Cholesterol in the prediction of atherosclerotic disease. New perspectives based on the Framingham Study. Annals of Internal Medicine 90, 85-91

Pocock, S.J., Shaper, A.G. and Phillips, A.N. (1989) Concentrations of high density lipoprotein cholesterol, triglyceride and total cholesterol in ischaemic heart disease. British Medical Journal 298, 998-1002

Bolibar, I. *et al.* (1995) Dose response relationships of serum lipid measurements with the extent of coronary stenosis. Strong, independent and comprehensive. Arteriosclerosis and Thrombosis 15, 1035-1042

The Multiple Risk Factor Intervention Trial

Stamler, J. Wentworth, D. and Neaton, J.D. (1986) Is the relationship between serum cholesterol and risk of premature death from coronary heart disease continuous or graded? Journal of American Medical Association 256, 2823-2828

The Scandinavian Simvastatin Survival Study (4S)

The Scandinavian Simvastatin Survival Study Group. Randomised trial of cholesterol lowering in 4444 patients with coronary heart disease: The Scandinavian Simvastatin Survival Study (4S). Lancet 345, 1274-5

The West of Scotland Study

Shepherd, J. *et al.* (1995) Prevention of coronary heart disease with pravastatin in men with hypercholesterolaemia New England Journal of Medicine 333, 1301-1307

4 The Lipoproteins

4.1 Introduction

The generally accepted definition of **lipids** is that of substances which are insoluble in aqueous media but soluble in non-polar organic solvents. This may often be qualified with the proviso that they are usually, but not exclusively, related to **fatty acids**. Fatty acids are long hydrocarbon chains, with or without double bonds, with terminal methyl and carboxyl groups. The specific nature of fatty acids will be discussed further in Chapter 7.

The major lipids found circulating in the blood are **cholesterol** and **cholesterol ester**, non-esterified fatty acids, **glycerophospholipids** and **triacylglycerol**. Some of these lipids, particularly free cholesterol and glycerophospholipids, are associated with the membranes of the various cells and platelets in the blood. However, all can also be found in the serum fraction. By their very nature these macromolecules cannot easily be transported in the aqueous environment of the blood, being insoluble except at very low concentrations. Two transport systems have been developed to overcome this problem. The first involves the binding of non-esterified fatty acids to the major serum protein, albumin. Fatty acids bind with varying levels of affinity to sites on the albumin molecule, rendering them relatively more soluble. Still, the capacity for transport of fatty acids in such a form is relatively low and the maximum concentrations which can be reached are approximately 2mM, after which increasing amounts of unbound fatty acid appear which can have severe toxic effects on the body.

Much more fatty acids can be transported esterified as triacylglycerol molecules. These highly hydrophobic neutral lipids are transported in the plasma inside the core of specific transport particles known as **lipoproteins**. Also found in the core of the lipoprotein particles are the other most hydrophobic of the lipids, cholesterol ester, which is cholesterol esterified to a fatty acid molecule. Cholesterol ester and triacylglycerol are protected from the aqueous environment by a coat of more hydrophilic lipids, i.e. glycerophospholipid (predominantly phosphatidylserine with lesser amounts of phosphatidylcholine and phosphtidylethanolamine) and free cholesterol. These molecule are arranged with their more hydrophobic regions oriented towards the core of the particles and their hydrophilic regions pointing outwards towards the plasma. The other major components of the lipoprotein particle are the proteins, or **apolipoproteins** as they are known. These represent a diverse collection of proteins of wide ranging structure and function. Some act to stabilise the structure of the particles and as such dip in and out of the lipid core anchoring the complex together. Others have functions such as receptor recognition and the activation or inhibition of specific enzymes. Some may display more than one of these functions. Minor components of the lipoproteins include the lipid soluble vitamins A, D, E and K and other lipid soluble compounds such as carotenoids and flavonoids.

Lipoproteins are generally spherical and span a range of sizes up to a maximum diameter of 1 μm. The physical properties of a lipoprotein particle are largely governed by the relative amounts of each component lipid while their metabolism is mainly directed by the presence of specific apolipoproteins. Figure 4.1 depicts the generalised structure of a lipoprotein particle.

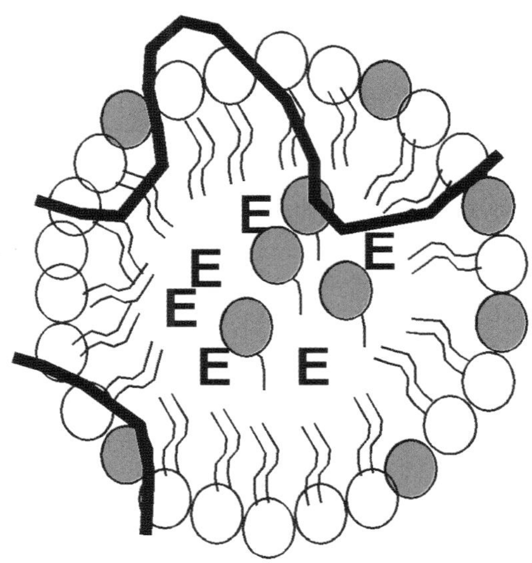

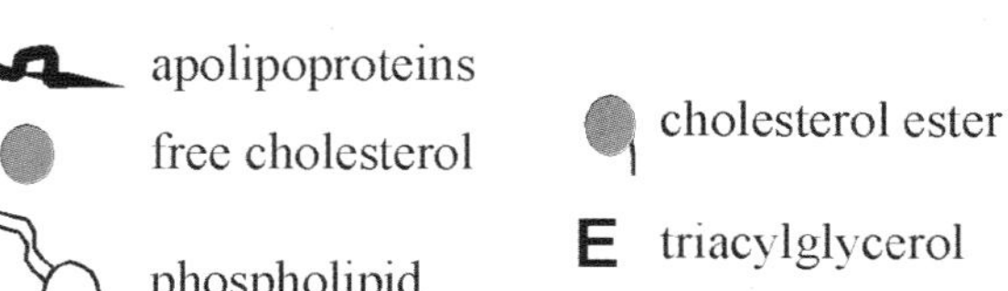

Figure 4.1
General overview of lipoprotein structure

4.2 The major lipoprotein classes

The presence of lipoproteins in the serum was first noted in 1929 when Machebeuf noted the presence of lipids, which co-precipitated with a protein fraction. However it was not until the 1940/50s that significant progress was made in the understanding of the nature of this material. It was quickly realised that the newly developed ultracentrifuge could be used to separate and analyse the lipoproteins. Under the intense gravitational field generated by this machine, lipoproteins could be separated by flotation depending on the background density of the surrounding medium. This led to the discovery that lipoproteins could be classified by their density (see table 4.1). In the plasma of a normal healthy individual, in the postprandial state, four major classes of lipoprotein are found; **chylomicrons**, **very low density lipoprotein (VLDL)**, **low density lipoprotein (LDL)** and **high density lipoprotein (HDL)**. If such an individual were subjected to an overnight fast then the chylomicrons would disappear from the serum. More detailed analysis of the HDL fraction has shown it to be clearly heterogeneous with at least two major sub-fractions, namely HDL_2 and HDL_3. As will be discussed later each of the lipoprotein classes exhibits some heterogeneity, which may be of considerable importance in their physiological and pathological functioning. In certain disease states other lipoprotein classes may become apparent such as **chylomicron remnants** and **intermediate density lipoprotein (IDL)**. These are normally rapidly cleared from the circulation and only accumulate when such clearance is impaired in some way. **Lipoprotein (a)** is another lipoprotein found in human blood. It actually represents a particle similar in composition to LDL but to which is attached an additional apolipoprotein known as Lp (a).

Table 4.1 Properties of the major lipoprotein classes

	Chylomicron	*VLDL*	*LDL*	*HDL*
Flotation (Sf)	>400	20-400	0-20	0-9
Density (g/ml)	0.95	<1.006	1.02-1.063	1.063-1.210
Size (nm)	>200	30-200	10-30	<10
Electrophoretic Mobility	None	pre-beta	Beta	alpha
Composition (%)				
Triacylglycerol	87	64-80	10	2-5
Total cholesterol	6	8-13	45	20
Phospholipids	4	6-15	25	30
Protein	1	8-10	20	48
Major apolipoproteins	B48,AI,AII, AIVCI, CII, CIII,E	AIV,B100, CI,CII, CIII,E	B100	AI,AII,AIV, CI,CII,CIII, D,E

4.3 Methods of separating lipoproteins

Understanding of the nature and metabolism of lipoproteins was greatly facilitated by the use of the **ultracentrifuge**. This machine allows the generation of extremely high gravitational forces by spinning samples in a vacuum. The earliest lipoprotein separations were performed in the analytical ultracentrifuge. Due to their lipid content lipoproteins can be made to "float" when subjected to the intense gravitational field generated in the ultracentrifuge, if the density of the surrounding solution is adjusted so that it is greater than that of the lipoprotein class to be separated. This is normally done by adding salts such as sodium chloride or sodium or potassium bromide. If the density of human serum is adjusted to 1.063g/ml then chylomicrons, VLDL, intermediate density lipoprotein (IDL) and LDL can all be separated in the analytical ultracentrifuge. As the samples are spinning each individual fraction sets up boundaries as it moves up the tube. The rate of movement of the boundaries can be optically determined and gives a measure of the density of a particular fraction. The width of the band containing the lipoprotein is directly related to its concentration in the serum.

While analytical ultracentrifugation is very useful in determining physical properties of a particular lipoprotein fraction it is technically difficult, requires expensive and specialist equipment and is time consuming. This technique has now been largely superseded by preparative ultracentrifugation. Based on the same principles, the preparative ultracentrifuge allows the isolation of individual lipoprotein so that their composition can be determined. Two major techniques are used namely; sequential flotation and density gradient separation. Sequential flotation usually employs a so-called fixed angle rotor that holds the sample tube at an angle of about 20-25°. The density of the sample is adjusted (again with salt solution) so that it is just above that of the lipoprotein fraction to be isolated. The sample is then spun in the ultracentrifuge and the lipoprotein fractions move to the top of the tube from where it can be collected. The density of the remaining sample is then further increased so that the next most dense fraction can be isolated and so on. Figure 4.2 show a schematic representation of how all the individual fractions may be isolated. A variant of this technique is density gradient ultracentrifugation. Using this method a continuous gradient of density is set up along the length of the ultracentrifuge tube. This is normally performed using a "swinging bucket" rotor where the tube spins in a horizontal position thus allowing the maximum possible "path-length". Each individual lipoprotein class then migrates to the position in the tube which represents it's own density. By carefully removing the sample from either the top or bottom of the tube each fraction can be collected.

While ultracentrifugation still represents the reference method for lipoprotein analysis, even separation in the preparative ultracentrifuge is relatively expensive and time consuming. For this reason a number of other techniques have been developed. **Electrophoresis**, usually on agarose gels, has proven a useful clinical diagnostic tool with lipoproteins migrating to characteristic regions as indicated in figure 4.3. Column chromatography, and more recently high performance

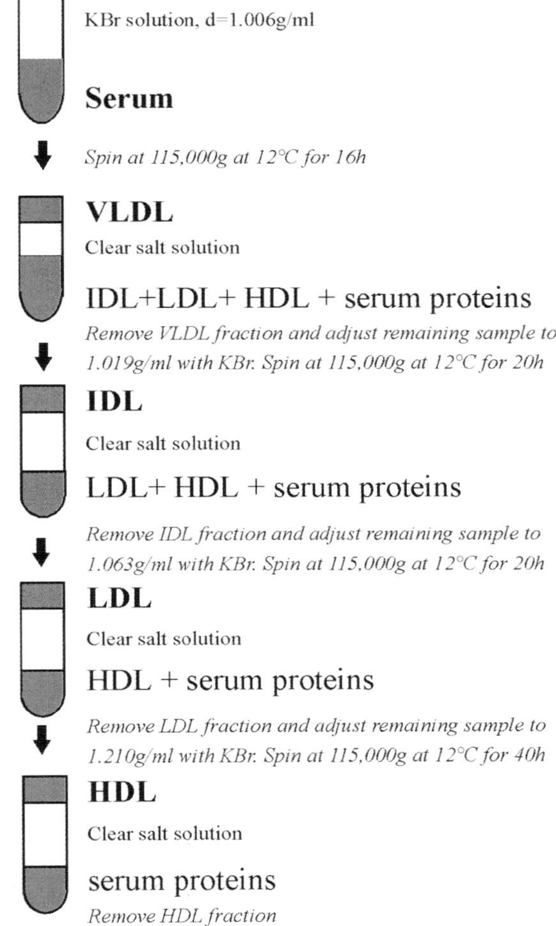

Figure 4.2
Scheme of separating lipoprotein in the preparative ultra-centrifuge using a fixed angle rotor

liquid chromatography, has proved useful for the separation of lipoproteins on the basis of size. However, one of the most important advances in elucidating the relationship of plasma lipoprotein concentrations to risk of coronary heart disease was the development of **precipitation techniques** for the isolation of HDL. These techniques are based on the fact that lipoproteins containing specific apolipoproteins (namely apoB and apoE) form insoluble complexes with some polyanionic compounds, in the presence of divalent cations. The most commonly used precipitants have been heparin, dextran sulphate and sodium phosphotungstate. Only the HDL fraction does not contain either of these apolipoproteins, thus after precipitation, this lipoprotein fraction is left in solution. On a fasting blood sample, determination of total serum cholesterol and supernatant (HDL) cholesterol allow the calculation, by difference, of the cholesterol content of the VLDL+LDL fraction. A further refinement is the use of the so-called Friedwall

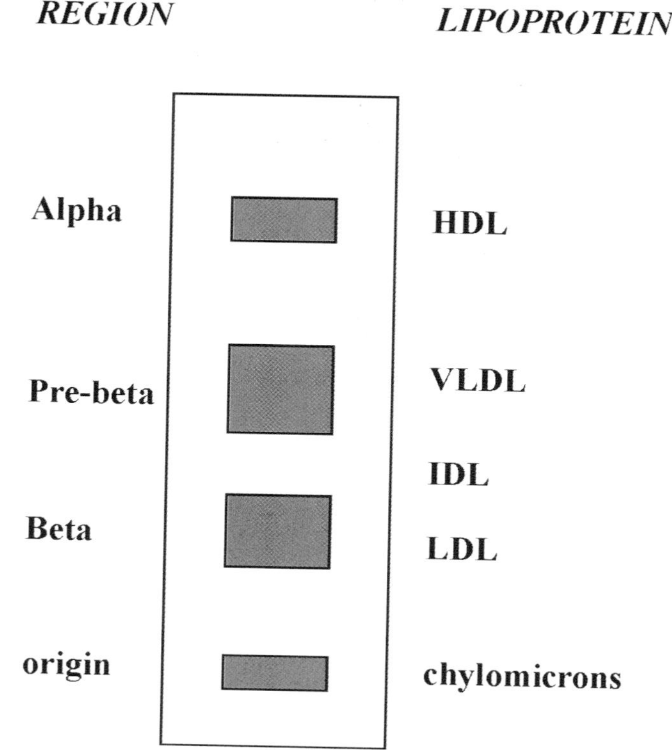

Figure 4.3 Electrophoretic separation of lipoproteins on agarose gels

equation to calculate LDL cholesterol concentration. This utilises the fact that, normally, the cholesterol content of the VLDL concentration is directly proportional to it's triacylglycerol content and that almost all of the triacylglycerol in the plasma is associated with VLDL. Thus, by measuring total plasma cholesterol and triacylglycerol (TAG) and HDL cholesterol (after precipitation) an estimate of LDL cholesterol can be determined as follows:

$$LDL\ chol = total\ chol - HDLchol - VLDL\ TAG/5$$

Some caution does have to be exercised in using this formula in patients with abnormal lipoprotein concentrations where the composition of the lipoproteins may be changed. Furthermore, most of the precipitation techniques for the separation of HDL do not work well with samples with elevated triacylglycerol concentrations. However, these rapid, easy and inexpensive techniques have allowed studies of large populations that were previously impractical using the ultracentrifuge.

4.5 Lipoprotein synthesis and secretion

The biosynthesis of lipids

The intestine

The major products of digestion of dietary fats are: fatty acids, 2-monoacylglycerol, lysoglycerophospholipids and free cholesterol. Once these have entered the enterocyte they are re-esterified to their original forms, namely: triacylglycerol, glycerophospholipids and cholesterol ester. Most of the triacylglycerol (about 85%) is formed from the re-esterification of 2-monoacyglycerol with fatty acids by the so-called **monoacyglycerol pathway**. Small amounts are formed from glycerol-3-phosphate by the **phosphatidic acid pathway** which will be described below. However the fatty acids first have to be activated by formation of their Coenzyme A derivatives.

$$R.COO^{-} + CoASH + ATP^{4-} \text{ ® } R.CO.SCoA + AMP^{2-} + PP_i^{3-}$$

This reaction is catalysed by *acyl-CoA synthetase* and the activated fatty acids produced are then added sequentially to the 2-monoacyglycerol to form diacyglycerol and then triacylglycerol by reactions catalysed by *acylglycerol palmitoyltransferase* and *diacylglycerol acyltransferase* respectively. Despite it's name the former enzyme can catalyse the addition of a number of long chain saturated and unsaturated fatty acids. In a similar way the additional fatty acid is esterified to the lysoglycerophospholipid to yield glycerophospholipid. A substantial proportion of the free cholesterol absorbed is re-esterified by the enzyme ***acyl CoA: cholesterol acyl transferase (ACAT)*** to form cholesterol ester. Triacylglycerol, phospholipid, cholesterol and cholesterol ester are all then combined with apolipoproteins to form chylomicrons.

The liver

The triacylglycerol which the liver deposits in VLDL particles can either come from cellular stores or be synthesised *de novo*. Recent evidence suggests that, even if stores within the hepatocytes are used they may first have to be hydrolysed and then reformed before being incorporated into the VLDL. Triacylglycerol synthesised *de novo* is formed via the **phosphatidic acid pathway** on the endoplasmic reticulum of the cell. The initial steps in this pathway are also common to the synthesis of glycerophospholipids. The first step involves the addition of a fatty acid (again from fatty acyl CoA) to the 1-position of the glycerol-3-phosphate to form 1-acylglycerophosphate (also called lysophosphatidate) by the action of *glycerophosphate acyltransferase* (figure 4.4).

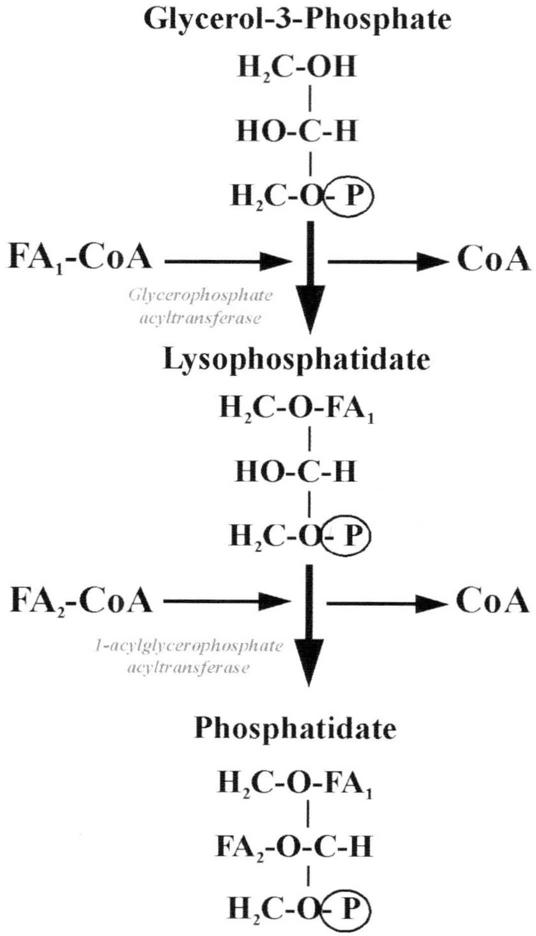

Glycerol-3-Phosphate

H_2C-OH
$HO-C-H$
$H_2C-O-(P)$

$FA_1-CoA \rightarrow$ ↓ $\rightarrow CoA$

Glycerophosphate acyltransferase

Lysophosphatidate

$H_2C-O-FA_1$
$HO-C-H$
$H_2C-O-(P)$

$FA_2-CoA \rightarrow$ ↓ $\rightarrow CoA$

1-acylglycerophosphate acyltransferase

Phosphatidate

$H_2C-O-FA_1$
$FA_2-O-C-H$
$H_2C-O-(P)$

Figure 4.4 Synthesis of phosphatidate

The enzyme *1-acylglycerophosphate acyltransferase* then catalyses the addition of a second fatty acid to the 2-position (figure 4.4). The phosphate group is then removed from the 3-position on the glycerol molecule by the action of the enzyme *phosphatidate phosphohydrolase* to form diacylglycerol (figure 4.5). This enzyme exists in both the cytoplasm and endoplasmic reticulum of the cell, but is only active on the latter. The cytoplasmic form of the enzyme appears to act as a potential pool of activity that can be translocated to the endoplasmic reticulum when triacylglycerol synthesis needs to be increased. One of the major stimuli for such translocation is an increase in intracelluar fatty acid concentrations. Finally, the enzyme, *diacylglycerol acyltransferase* catalyses the addition of a third fatty acid to the 3-position of the diacylglycerol (figure 4.6).

Glycerophospholipids can be synthesised by several routes. One involves the formation of cytidine diphosphodiacylgycerol (CDP-

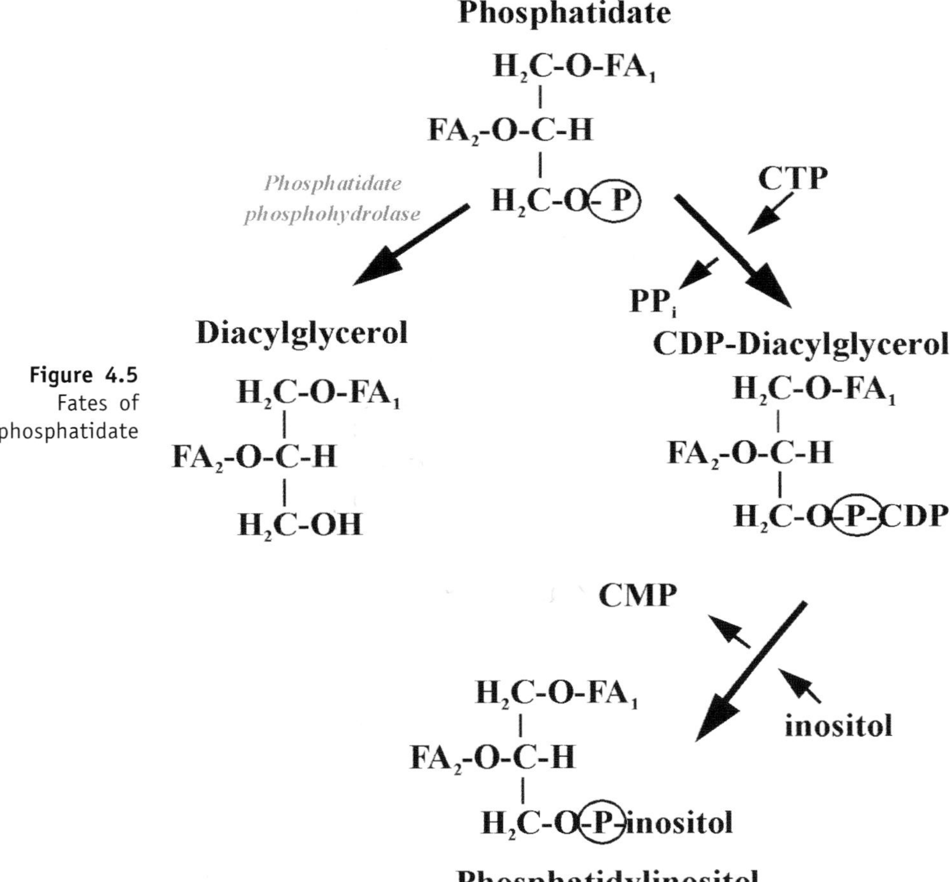

Figure 4.5 Fates of phosphatidate

diacylglycerol) (figure 4.5). This activated phosphatidyl unit then reacts with an alcohol group (such as inositol) to form the glycerophospholipid (such as phosphatidylinositol). Alternatively, glycerophospholipids may be formed from diacylglycerol through interaction with an alcohol, activated by the addition of a CDP molecule (e.g. CDP-choline, CDP-ethanolamine) (figure 4.6).

Cholesterol incorporated into VLDL can also come from either intracellular stores or de novo synthesis. Cholesterol is synthesised from acetyl CoA. The rate limiting step in the synthesis of cholesterol is the conversion of 3-hydroxy-3-methyl-glutaryl Coenzyme A (HMGCoA) to mevalonate as catalyzed by the enzyme ***HMGCoA reductase***. Regulation of the activity of this enzyme will be discussed later.

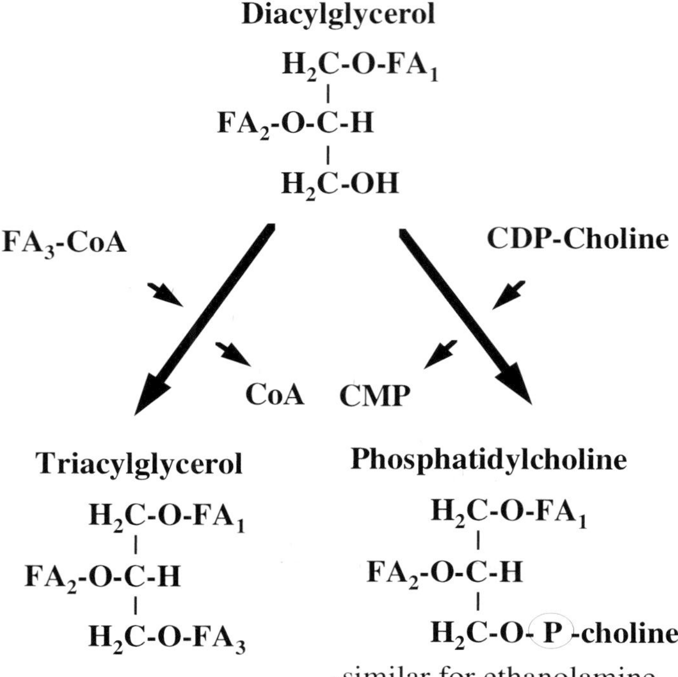

Figure 4.6
Fates of Diacylglycerol

Assembly and secretion of the lipoproteins

The major organs involved in the synthesis and secretion of lipoproteins are the intestine and the liver. The intestine produces chylomicrons and the liver VLDL. Both organs produce components of HDL but the particle is probably assembled in the blood and interstitial fluid and will be considered separately below (section 4.6). Most of our knowledge of the processes involved in the assembly of lipoproteins and their ultimate secretion is based on studies of the liver and, in particular, hepatocytes in culture. However, it seems likely that the general principles are similar for the assembly of chylomicrons in the intestine though the regulation of these processes is likely to be different.

The assembly of the lipoprotein particle starts with the synthesis of the major apolipoprotein, **apoB$_{48}$** in the chylomicron and **apoB$_{100}$** in VLDL. These two proteins are actually the product of the same gene and apoB$_{48}$ is produced in the intestine by specific editing of the apoB mRNA such that only 48% of the whole protein is produced. Translation of the mRNA results in the production of a signal peptide, which directs the ribosome carrying the mRNA and growing apoB molecule to the rough endoplasmic reticulum. Synthesis of the protein then continues and the emerging peptide enters the lumen of the endoplasmic reticulum. As it grows the protein folds in a particular confirmation held in position by disulphide bridges. This folding is essential for the further assembly of the lipoprotein particle. At this point, the emerging apoB molecule has one of two possible fates; either it can go on to be incorporated into a lipoprotein particle or it can be degraded. The deciding factor as to which path it follows is the addition of triacylglycerol to the protein. If no triacylglycerol is added then the protein follows a degradatory pathway with only a small terminal peptide ultimately being secreted. If triacylglycerol is added then translation of the apoB continues and the lipoprotein particle matures. Thus, lipoprotein production is regulated by the availability of the lipid. It may seem wasteful to degrade the apoB without the protein ever serving a useful purpose but this mechanism has probably evolved to allow the cell to respond to rapidly changes that may occur in the influx of fatty acids.

The addition of triacylglycerol to the apoB requires the action of a transfer protein known as the **microsomal triglyceride transfer protein (MTP)**. MTP is a hetero-dimer consisting of two subunits. The smaller subunit is identical to the enzyme, *protein disulphide isomerase* and it's exact function remains uncertain. The larger subunit possess the lipid transfer activity. Our understanding of the actions of this protein have been increased considerably by the finding that the rare genetic disease hypobetalipoproteinemia, where apoB containing lipoproteins are absent from the plasma, results from a lack of functional MTP. Such patients are unable to absorb dietary lipids or lipid soluble vitamins.

With it's load of triacylglygerol, the apoB molecules continues to be translated and aquires other lipids including cholesterol, cholesterol ester and phospholipid. Once the full-length apoB has been formed it is finally released into the lumen of the endoplasmic reticulum. At this point, it probably moves into the smooth endoplasmic reticulum where the bulk of the lipid is added to the particle, without a requirement for MTP. The particle undergoes further maturation as it passes through the Golgi apparatus finally to emerge as a spherical lipoprotein particle ready for secretion. The main features of this pathway are indicated in figure 4.7.

4.6 The lipoprotein pathways

The transport of lipids around the body in lipoproteins can be conveniently divided into three major pathways; the exogenous pathway, the endogenous pathway and the reverse cholesterol transport pathway. The exogenous pathway is associated with the distribution of lipids of dietary origin from the intestine to the rest of the tissues. The endogenous pathway is associated with the transport of lipids of hepatic origin and the reverse cholesterol transport pathway is associated with the transport of cholesterol from peripheral tissue to the liver.

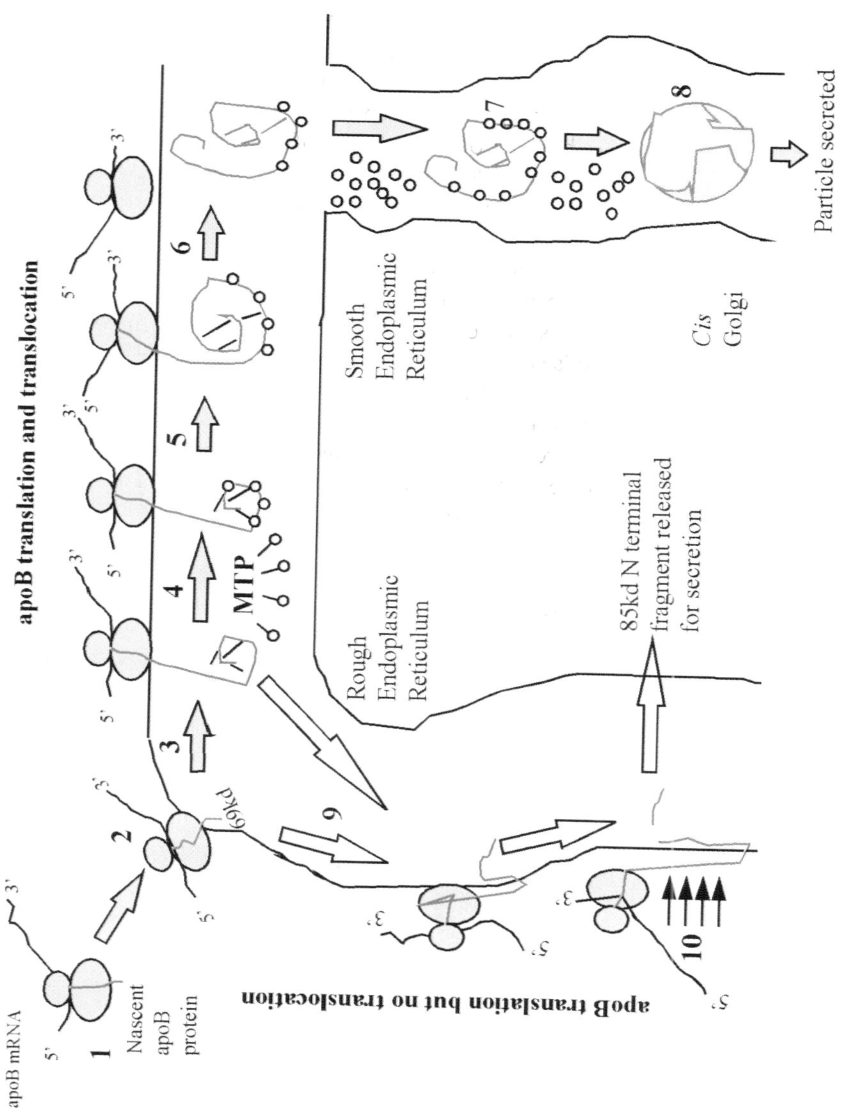

Figure 4.7
Lipoprotein assembly

(1) initiation of translation of apoB, (2) translation and translocation of apoB into the rough endoplasmic reticulum, (3) folding of the N-terminal of apoB, (4) Addition of triacylglycerol and cholesterol ester by MTP, (5) Continued translation and translocation of apoB, (6) formation of a lipid poor lipoprotein, (7) addition of bulk lipid, (8) assembly and secretion of mature lipoprotein, (9) translation but arrested translocation of apoB in the absence of triacylglycerol, (10) degradation of apoB.

The exogenous pathway

A summary of the Exogenous Pathway is shown in figure 4.8. The chylomicron particle is secreted from the enterocyte into lymph vessels. The particles then pass, *via* the thoracic duct, into the bloodstream at the level of the jugular vein. The particles are exceptionally rich in triacylglycerol and the major protein component is apoB_{48}. On entering the blood stream the particles immediately undergo important changes in their apolipoprotein composition. They gain apoCs and apoE *via* exchange from circulating HDL particles. The acquisition of **apoC-II** is particularly important for the further metabolism of the chylomicron particle. This protein appears to mediate the interaction of the chylomicron with the enzyme ***lipoprotein lipase***. This enzyme is produced by a variety of tissues, quantitatively most important being adipose tissue and muscle. The protein migrates from its site of synthesis and is found anchored, *via* polysaccharide chains, to the capillary walls within the tissue. This enzyme is a glycoprotein and is one of a family of related triacylglycerol *lipases* which includes the digestive enzyme, *pancreatic lipase* and the liver specific enzyme, ***hepatic triglyceride lipase***. Activated by the apoC-II on the surface of the chylomicron, LPL hydrolyses the fatty acids from the 1(3) position of the particles triacylglycerol molecules, yielding fatty acids and monoacylglycerol. Monoacylglycerol may be further metabolised to produce free fatty acid and glycerol. It was originally thought that virtually all the fatty acids released through the action of LPL were taken up locally by the tissues, i.e. muscle or adipose tissue. However, more recent evidence suggests that appreciable amounts may escape local uptake and be released into the circulation.

As the triacylglycerol is hydrolysed the chylomicron particle "shrinks". The loss of core lipid makes an increasing proportion of the surface material (phospholipid, free cholesterol and protein) redundant and this is shed from the particle. It is believed that much of this material is taken up by other lipoproteins, particularly HDL. Eventually, the chylomicron loses it's apoCII content and can no longer maintain LPL activity. The resultant particle depleted in triacylglycerol and much reduced in size is called a chylomicron remnant. These particles, while still containing some triacylglycerol are relatively enriched in cholesterol ester. Remnants are normally rapidly removed from the circulation by the liver and do not accumulated in any quantity in plasma. However, in type III hyperlipidaemia (see chapter 5) they do accumulate and are believed to be associated with an increased risk of atherosclerosis found in such patients. A number of pathways appear to be involved in the removal of chylomicron remants by the liver. The **LDL receptor** (see below) may bind and internalise chylomicron remnants but it is not essential for effective clearance. This is shown in those suffering from familial hypercholesterolaemia who, despite lacking functional LDL

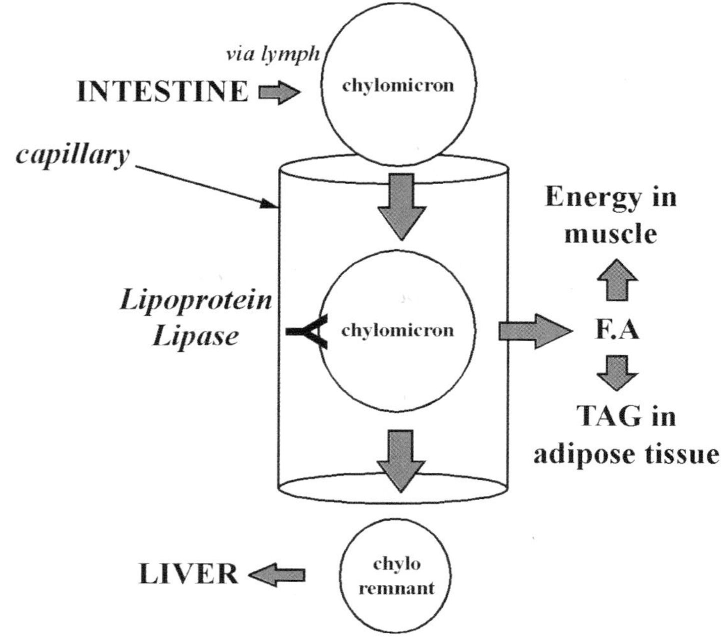

Figure 4.8 Overview of the exogenous lipoprotein pathway

See text for details

receptors have normal plasma concentrations of chylomicron remnants. The uptake of chylomicrons by the liver is mediated by **apolipoprotein E** and a receptor with considerable homology to the LDL receptor, the **low density lipoprotein receptor -related protein (LRP)**, may well play an important role in mediating this uptake. However, recent evidence also indicates that *hepatic triglyceride lipase* may play an important role in mediating the binding of the chylomicron remnant to the LRP. Further research is obviously required to fully elucidate the processes by which chylomicron remnants are cleared from the circulation. Once taken into the cell the chylomicron remnant particles are degraded in lysosome and the lipids released into the hepatocytes for further metabolism.

The endogenous pathway

A summary of the Endogenous Pathway is shown in figure 4.9. The endogenous lipoprotein pathway represents the route whereby lipids secreted from the liver are distributed around the body. The pathway starts with the assembly of VLDL as outlined earlier. VLDL particles are secreted directly into the blood stream and as seen in table 4.1 are, like chylomicrons, triacylglycerol-rich. The major apolipoprotein is $apoB_{100}$ and the particles contain lesser amounts of apoE and apoCs. On entering the plasma the content of the two latter proteins increases further due to transfer from HDL. Like chylomicrons, VLDL represent

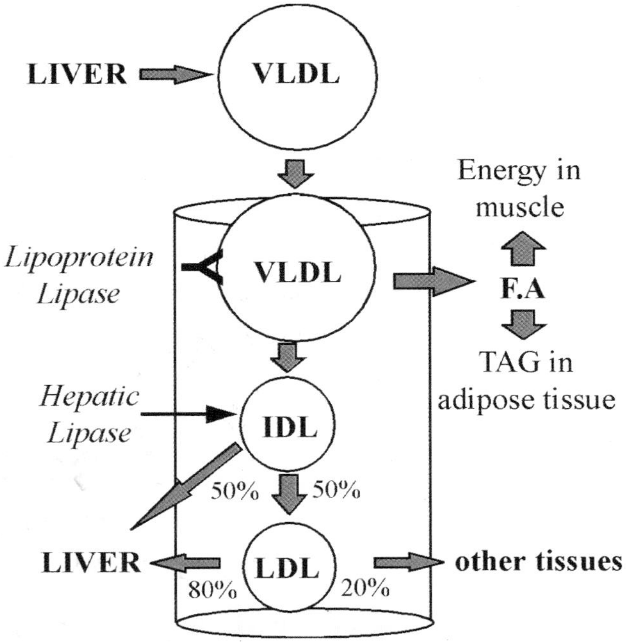

Figure 4.9 Overview of the endogenous lipoprotein pathway

See text for details

substrates for the action of lipoprotein lipase. LPL is again activated by the presence of apoCII on the particle and the fatty acids released are taken up for energy storage (adipose tissue) or production (muscle) in the same way as from chylomicrons. Thus, both chylomicrons and VLDL follow a similar route of metabolism. However, it is important to note that plasma concentrations of the two lipoproteins and indeed, the activity of LPL in different tissues will vary depending on the metabolic circumstances. For example, following a mixed meal containing a significant amount of fat, the plasma concentration of chylomicrons will be relatively high. In addition, assuming a significant amount of carbohydrate in the meal, plasma insulin concentration are also likely to be high. Insulin, stimulates the activity of LPL in adipose tissue and thus, much of the dietary fatty acids will be directed towards storage in adipose tissue. By contrast, after an overnight fast few, if any, chylomicrons will be entering the circulation and plasma insulin concentrations will be low. In this condition VLDL will be the predominant triacylglycerol -rich lipoprotein and LPL activity will be relatively high in muscle. Thus significantly more fatty acids, now of endogenous origin, will be directed toward energy production in muscle.

The remnant particles produced after hydrolysis of most of the triacylglycerol core, of the VLDL, are termed intermediate density lipoproteins (IDL). These particles, which have lost most of their apolipoproteins apart from apoB100 and apoE, can follow one of two routes. They can be removed by the liver following the interaction of apoE with the LDL receptor (see below) or they can remain in the plasma and be converted to low density lipoprotein (LDL) particles with the loss of apoE. The mechanism whereby IDL is converted to LDL has not been fully elucidated but it probably involves further lipolysis by *lipoprotein lipase* and, as the particle becomes smaller, by *hepatic triglyceride lipase*. The relative amount of IDL that follows these two pathways varies substantially between species. In the rat most of the IDL is directly removed by the liver and as a result this species has very low amounts of circulating LDL. By contrast, in the human only about half the IDL is removed directly with the remainder forming the considerable amounts of LDL which is found in the human circulation. LDL is then removed from the circulation after binding to LDL receptors either in the liver or in extrahepatic tissues. The LDL receptor shows a lower affinity for LDL (which contains only apoB) than for IDL (with which the receptor interacts through apoE). Approximately 80% of plasma LDL is removed by the liver while the other 20% is removed by all the other tissues of the body combined. LDL is then taken into the cell by the process known as the LDL receptor pathway.

LDL receptor pathway

The LDL receptor is a glycoprotein expressed on the plasma membrane of most cell types in the body. It's existence and the pathway through which it's expression is regulated was first elucidated by the pioneering experiments of Goldstein and Brown in the 1970s using cultured human fibroblasts. They demonstrated that the underlying defect in familial hypercholesterolaemia was an absence or impairment of function in the LDL receptor (chapter 5). Figure 4.10 shows the basic structure of the LDL receptor. It consists of five domains. The N-terminal end contains the ligand binding domain. This is an area rich in cysteine residues and multiple loops. It contains clusters of negatively charged amino acids through which the receptor interacts with positively charged regions of $apoB_{100}$ and apoE. The second domain shows a high degree of homology to the extracellular domain of the protein precursor to epidermal growth factor, perhaps suggesting evolution from a common gene. This is followed by a highly glycosylated region just prior to a membrane spanning domain which anchors the receptor in the membrane. Finally, there is a short C-terminal cytoplasmic domain.

The LDL receptor will bind a number of $apoB_{100}$ or apoE containing ligands including; chylomicron remnants, IDL and LDL itself. Receptors are located in specific regions of the membrane known as **coated pits**. These make up about 2% of the cell surface and are rich in a protein called **clathrin**. This protein produces a highly ordered structure of pentagons and hexagons in the form of a lattice along the cytoplasmic surface of the membrane. The polymerisation of clathrin is thought to

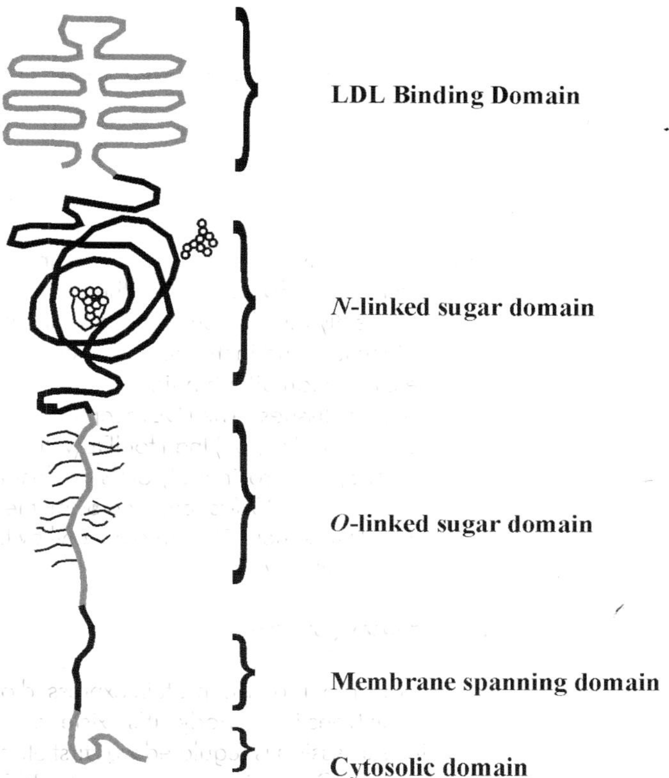

Figure 4.10 Structure of the LDL receptor

be responsible for the "pinching off" of regions of the membranes and the internalisation of "coated vesicles". The lipoprotein particles, bound to their receptors are located in the centre of these vesicles. The clathrin coat is then lost and each vesicle is now termed an endosome. A drop of pH inside the vesicle results in the uncoupling of receptor and ligand. A receptor-rich region of these endosomes then buds off and recycles the receptors to the plasma membrane. This process is, however, not 100% efficient and a proportion of the receptor is lost during each cycle. Thus if a cell is to maintain a constant level of receptor expression it must also be synthesising new receptors to replace those lost. In the absence of such synthesis the number of receptors will fall and LDL uptake diminish. The remaining portion of the endosome fuses with a lysosome to form a secondary lysosome where the lipoprotein particles are degraded. The apolipoprotein is broken down by proteases to release the free amino acids, the cholesterol ester to free cholesterol (and fatty acid) and any remaining triacylglycerol to free fatty acids and glycerol.

As most of the ligands for the LDL receptor are cholesterol-rich, one of the major consequences of lipoprotein uptake is an accumulation of intracellular cholesterol. Cholesterol is however potentially toxic to the cell and a number of mechanisms exist to prevent it's over-accumulation. First of all the activity ACAT is stimulated. This enzyme is responsible for the intracellular conversion of free cholesterol to the more inert cholesterol ester form. Cholesterol ester can be stored, within the cell, in relatively high concentrations with little deleterious effects on the cell. Secondly, an over-accumulation of cholesterol leads to the down-regulation of expression of the LDL receptor gene. As already indicated recycling of receptors is incomplete so, reduced expression of the gene will ultimately reduce the number of cell surface receptors and thereby inhibit the further uptake of more cholesterol-rich lipoproteins. The third level of regulation is exerted on the cell's ability to synthesise cholesterol *de novo*. Most cells in the body have the capacity to synthesise enough cholesterol for their own needs. If excess cholesterol is supplied through the action of the LDL receptor then the synthetic capacity of the cell is reduced. This regulation is exerted at the level of the enzyme HMGCoA reductase. Thus if cellular cholesterol concentrations increase, HMGCoA reductase gene expression is inhibited and the cell shuts down it's cholesterol synthetic capacity. In summary over-accumulation of cholesterol in a cell, due to uptake *via* the LDL receptor, increases cholesterol esterification, inhibits the production of new LDL receptors and inhibits the cells capacity to make cholesterol. The major details of this pathway are illustrated in figure 4.11.

Regulation of gene expression by cholesterol

One of the primary findings of Goldstein and Brown was that cholesterol appears to have the ability to regulate the production of proteins directly involved in lipoprotein metabolism. As already discussed above this include *HMGCoA reductase* and the LDL receptor. Other proteins found to be regulated by intracelluar cholesterol concentrations include; *HMGCoA synthase, cholesterol 7–alpha hydroxylase* and possibly, *MTP*. The mechanism by which cholesterol exerts such regulation has been the subject of intensive research. It is now clear that the production of these protein is regulated by cholesterol at the level of gene expression. The promoters of these genes contain sequences which code for regions known as **sterol regulatory elements** (SREs). These act as binding sites for specific proteins termed **sterol regulatory element binding proteins** (SREBPs). For example, the expression of the LDL receptor gene appears to be regulated by the 125kDa protein, SREBP-1. This protein is found bound to the endoplasmic reticulum and nuclear membranes. If the concentration of sterol in the cell drops, then the protein is proteolytically cleaved to generate a 68kDa fraction which migrates to the nucleus and activates transcription of the LDL receptor

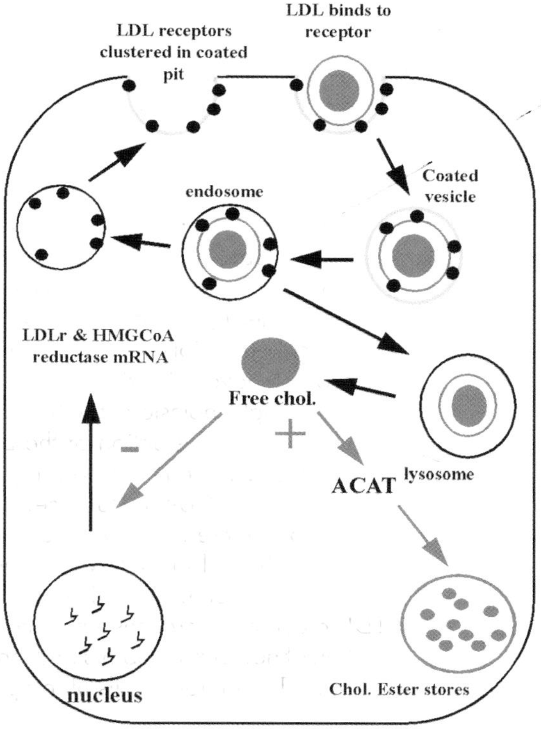

Figure 4.11
The LDL receptor pathway

See text for details

gene. When sterol concentrations rise proteolysis of the 125kDa protein is inhibited and transcription is down-regulated. It is also of note that this regulation is not brought about by cholesterol itself but by oxygenated derivatives. If cultured cells are incubated with pure cholesterol then no regulatory effect is seen. However, if the oxygenated sterol, 25-hydroxy-cholesterol is used instead then this will effectively down-regulate LDL receptor activity. Other genes, such as MTP, appear to have modified SREs in their promoters such that increased levels of sterol may actually increase gene expression.

The LDL receptor family

The LDL receptor is only one of a family of closely -related cell surface lipoprotein receptors. These include the LDL receptor related receptor (LRP) and the more recently discovered VLDL receptor.

The LDL receptor –related protein

As it's name suggests the LDL receptor–related protein (LRP) is a receptor displaying considerable homology to the LDL receptor itself. It is expressed in high levels in the liver, brain and placenta and is able to mediate the cellular uptake of apoE containing lipoproteins including chylomicron remnants and IDL. It has been postulated to play an important role in the rapid hepatic removal of such remnant particles from the circulation. Unlike the LDL receptor it does not recognise apoB. The interaction of apoE with the LRP may be modulated by the apoCIII content of the lipoprotein particles as the presence of high amount of apoCIII appears to inhibit binding. As well as a role in mediating hepatic remnant removal, the LRP has been suggested to play a role in uptake of lipoproteins by macrophages during the atherosclerotic process. Like the scavenger receptors the LRP also binds a range of polyanionic non-lipoprotein ligands.

A 323 amino acid polypeptide, called receptor-associated polypeptide (**RAP**) has been discovered which effectively competes with all known ligands for binding to the LRP. RAP is synthesised on the endoplasmic reticulum but is not secreted from the cell. It has been suggested that RAP may play a role in regulating LRP expression by binding to LRP within recycling vesicles within cells and preventing the return of the receptor to the plasma membrane.

The VLDL receptor

The most recently discovered member of the lipoprotein receptor family is the **VLDL receptor**. Like the LRP, the VLDL receptor is highly homologous to the LDL receptor but has a different expression pattern. It is highly transcribed in heart, skeletal muscle and adipose tissue. Again like the LRP, it binds apoE, but not apoB, containing lipoproteins and ligand binding is inhibited by RAP. The function of the VLDL receptor remains to be elucidated but it's localisation and ligand specificity has led to the suggestion that it may be involved in binding of triacylglycerol –rich lipoproteins, thereby facilitating the delivery of fatty acids to the tissues.

The macrophage scavenger receptors

The **macrophage scavenger receptors** represent yet another discovery of Goldstein and Brown. In studying the potential mechanisms whereby **macrophages** take-up LDL to become foam cells in the artery wall, they showed that this was not mediated by the "classical" LDL receptor, but by an alternative uncontrolled receptor pathway. They found that macrophage scavenger receptor activity can mediate the uptake of vast amounts of chemically modified LDL. Early experiments showed that while native LDL did not interact with these receptors, LDL in which the apoB moiety had been acetylated bound avidly. More recently, it has been shown that oxidation of LDL (see chapter 6) also produces particles which are recognised by the scavenger receptors. It is now generally accepted that such modification of the LDL is an important step in the atherosclerotic process. Cloning studies have indicated that there are two isoforms of the scavenger receptor, type I and type II which are produced from a single gene by alternative splicing of the mRNA. These receptors do not only bind modified LDL but also act as binding sites for some polyribonucleotides, some polysaccharides, such as dextran sulphate and anionic phospholipids such as phosphatidylserine.

Reverse cholesterol transport

Reverse cholesterol transport is the pathway by which cholesterol can be removed from peripheral cells and deposited in the liver. In the liver such cholesterol can undergo a number of possible fates including; storage as cholesterol ester; re-incorporation into VLDL and secretion back into the circulation. Alternatively, it can be secreted in the bile as either free cholesterol or after conversion to bile acids. Incomplete reabsorption of free cholesterol and bile acids within the intestine represents the primary route of cholesterol excretion.

Reverse cholesterol transport is the primary function of HDL. Classically, HDL has been divided into two major subfractions; HDL_2 and HDL_3. HDL_2 is the least dense (HDL_2, 1.063-1.0125g/ml vs HDL_3, 1.125-1.210) and larger of the two fractions. In fact, HDL_2 itself consists of two distinguishable subfraction HDL_{2b} (density; 1.063-1.10g/ml) and HDL_{2a} (1.10-1.125g/ml). However, HDL particles also exhibit heterogenity in terms of their apoliporotein content. While the majority of HDL particles contain both **apolipoprotein AI** and **apoAII** a subpopulation of particles, ranging from 11-45% of the total, contain apoAI alone. The relative importance of these two types of particle in the reverse cholesterol transport pathways remains to be established. In addition to these "mature" spherical HDL particles much smaller amounts of other apoAI containing particles can be found in the plasma. One is called pre-ß-1 HDL (based on it's electrophoretic mobility) and the other are pre-ß-2 HDL. Pre-ß-1 HDL makes up about 2-5% of the entire HDL population. They are small (molecular mass of about 60-70kDa) particles which contain apoAI associated with fairly low amounts (10-40%) of lipid, primarily phospholipid. Pre-ß-2 HDL are discoidal in shape, represent 2-3% of the total HDL population and contain apoAI, phospholipid and some free cholesterol.

The precise role of each of these types of HDL in reverse cholesterol transport remains to be elucidated but the following model is based on suggestions by Fielding and Fielding (1995). ApoAI is produced by both the liver and the intestine. It is secreted into the plasma as a 249 amino acid propeptide but is rapidly cleaved by proteases to yield the mature 243 amino acid protein. In the plasma, free apoAI probably rapidly associates with phospholipid to form pre-ß-1 HDL. Pre-ß-1

HDL interacts with peripheral cells to remove free cholesterol. The nature of this interaction remains to be fully elucidated, but may involve the active transport of cholesterol to the plasma membrane of the cells and its transfer to pre-ß-1 HDL following the binding of the HDL to specific receptor site. Some evidence suggests that such binding may initiate a cell signalling pathway, possibly involving *protein kinase* C, which stimulates the further movement of cholesterol to the cell membrane. Studies utilising radio-labelled cholesterol indicate that once incorporated into pre-ß-1 HDL, cholesterol is quickly transferred to pre-ß-2 HDL. The most likely explanation for this is that a number of pre-ß-1 particle fuse together to create the larger pre-ß-2 particle.

The next step in the reverse cholesterol transport pathway is the attachment of the enzyme, ***lecithin: cholesterol acyl transferase*** (**LCAT**) to the pre-ß-2 HDL particle. LCAT esterifies free cholesterol by removing a fatty acid from the 2-position of phosphatidylcholine and esterifying it to the free hydroxyl group of free cholesterol molecules. This creates a highly hydrophobic molecule which then migrates to the centre of the lipoprotein particle. It is the move of cholesterol ester into the core of the lipoprotein which converts the discoidal pre-ß-2 particles into "mature" spherical HDL particles. The initial spherical particle to be formed is probably HDL_3. The latter lipoprotein continues to accept cholesterol, partly from the redundant surface component of chylomicrons and VLDL as they are acted upon by lipoprotein lipase, and perhaps through further interaction with peripheral cells. The cholesterol is again esterified by LCAT and, as the particle grows, it enters the HDL_2 density ranges. The lipoprotein now loses its affinity for LCAT and the enzyme is released. The next step is to deliver the cholesterol ester load to the liver. Two major pathways for such clearance have been described. The first is a direct interaction of HDL_2 with liver cells. The HDL is recognised by specific binding sites on the surface of hepatocytes and thereby delivers it's load of cholesterol ester. As the particle shrinks it re-enters the density range of HDL_3 density range and re-circulates in the plasma taking up and esterifying more cholesterol. The exact molecular mechanisms whereby HDL interacts with the liver remain to be fully elucidated. The second pathway is *via* the transfer of cholesterol ester to less dense lipoprotein fractions. This transfer is mediated by the circulating protein; **cholesterol ester transfer protein (CETP)**. This catalyses the exchange of neutral lipids between lipoproteins. Cholesterol ester may be transferred to chylomicron remnants or VLDL in exchange for triacylglycerol. The cholesterol may then be returned to the liver through the subsequent uptake of chylomicron remnant, IDL and LDL. It has been suggested that the major role of CETP is not, however associated with reverse cholesterol transport, but with the cycling of free cholesterol from LDL to HDL. This cholesterol is then esterified and then returned to LDL, in exchange for more free cholesterol. The purpose of this shuttling of cholesterol between LDL and HDL and the relative importance of CETP in the reverse cholesterol transport pathway remains to be established. Interestingly, the rat, which expresses very little CETP, is relatively resistant to atherosclerosis. Figure 4.12 shows an overview of the Reverse Cholesterol Transport Pathway.

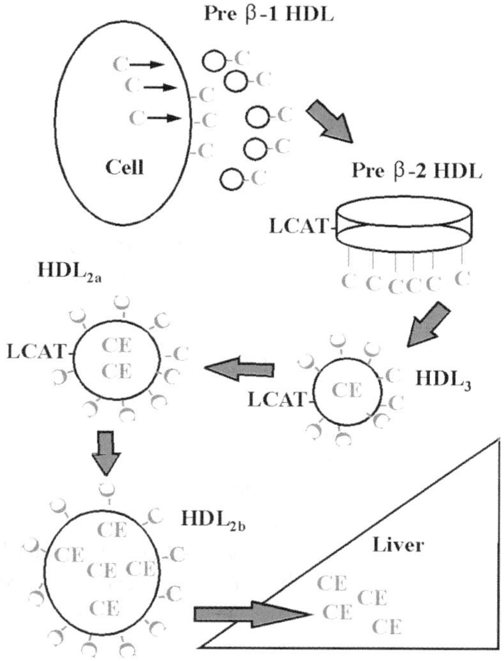

Figure 4.12

Reverse cholesterol transport
Cholesterol (C)
Cholesterol ester (CE)

(See text for details)

Lipoprotein (a)

Considerable interest exists in lipoprotein (a) due to it's apparent association with increased risk of coronary heart disease. As described in section 4.2, lipoprotein (a) consists of an LDL -like particle with additional protein attached known as apo (a). Apo (a) has been shown to exhibit a marked structural homology to plasminogen, a protein involved in the coagulation and fibrinolytic system. The metabolism of this lipoprotein is still poorly understood but it appears that apo (a) is produced by the liver and probably associates with LDL in the circulation. Concentrations of lipoprotein (a) vary markedly between individuals and this is associated with the considerable genetic variation, which produces apo (a) of a variety of different sizes, rather than differences in metabolic factors. A number of studies have demonstrated a link between plasma lipoprotein (a) concentrations and increased risk of coronary heart disease but this may also dependent on prevailing LDL cholesterol concentrations as well.

4.7 Conclusions

Lipoproteins represent an important mechanism whereby lipids can be freely circulated around the body. Their unique physical characteristics have led to the development of a range of techniques for their separation. As these techniques have been developed so has our understanding of their metabolism and their role in atherosclerosis. It is now clear that the apolipoproteins play an important role in directing the metabolism of the different lipoprotein classes through their modulation of enzyme activities and as ligands for different receptors. LDL represents the major cholesterol carrying lipoprotein in human plasma but its uptake by most of the cells of the body is carefully regulated. However, when LDL becomes oxidised in the artery wall then a separate receptor pathway leads to its uncontrolled uptake by macrophages and the formation of foam cells. In contrast, HDL appears to protect the artery wall from the development of atherosclerosis, in part, through its role in the reverse cholesterol transport pathway.

Key references

Lipoprotein synthesis and secretion

Kent, C. (1995) Eucaryotic phospholipid biosynthesis. Annual Reviews of Biochemistry. 64, 315-343

Davis, R.A. and Vance, J.E. (1996) Structure assembly and secretion of lipoproteins. In: Biochemistry of Lipids, Lipoproteins and Memebranes (Edited by D.E. Vance & J. Vance) New Comprehensive Biochemistry Volume 31. Elsevier 473-493

White, D.A. *et al.* (1998) The assembly of triacylglycerol-rich lipoproteins: an essential role for the microsomal triacylglycerol transfer protein. British Journal of Nutrition 80, 219-229

Lipoprotein pathways

Havel, R. (1997) Postprandial lipid metabolism: an overview.Proceedings of the Nutrition Society 56, 659-666

Fielding, P.E. and Fielding, C.J. (1996) Dynamics of lipoprotein transport in the human circulatory system (1996) In: Biochemistry of Lipids, Lipoproteins and Membranes (Edited by D.E. Vance & J. Vance) New Comprehensive Biochemistry Volume 31. Elsevier 495-515

Lipoprotein receptors

Brown, M.S. & Goldstein, J.L. (1986) A receptor mediated pathway for cholesterol homeostasis. Science 232, 34-47

Krieger, M. and Herz, J. (1994) Structure and functions of multiligand liporotein receptors: Macrophage scavenger receptor and LDL receptor -related protein (LRP). Annual Reviews of Biochemistry 63, 601-638

Schneider, W.J. (1996) Removal of lipoproteins from plasma. In: Biochemistry of Lipids, Lipoproteins and Membranes (Edited by D.E. Vance & J. Vance) New Comprehensive Biochemistry Volume 31. Elsevier 517-541

Reverse cholesterol transport

Fielding, C.J. & Fielding, P.E. (1995) Molecular physiology of reverse cholesterol transport. Journal of Lipid Research 36, 311-228

Oram, J.F. and Yokoyama, S. (1996) Apolipoprotein-mediated removal of cellular cholesterol and phospholipids. Journal of Lipid Research. 37, 2473-2491

Lipoprotein (a)

Hajjar, K.A. and Nachman, R.L. (1996) The role of lipoprotein (a) in atherogenesis and thrombosis. Annual Reviews of Medicine. 47, 423-442

5 Hyperlipoproteinaemias

5.1 Introduction

The study of diseases in which lipoproteins are increased in the blood (hyperlipoproteinaemias) has provided much of our understanding of coronary heart disease. For example, the observation of high levels of cholesterol found in plasma of patients with **familial hypercholesterolaemia** led to the hypothesis that high plasma cholesterol is a risk factor for coronary heart disease (discussed in chapter 3).

The first descriptions of hyperlipoproteinaemias were based upon measurement of cholesterol and triacylglycerol (TAG) in the plasma. A more comprehensive classification, described by **Fredrickson**, in 1972, was that based upon the separation of lipoproteins by electrophoresis. The World Health Organisation (WHO) adopted Fredrickson's classification of hyperlipoproteinaemias according to the plasma lipoprotein profile. The lipoprotein phenotypes, as the different lipoprotein profiles are termed, are shown in table 5.1. Classification of hyperlipoproteinaemias in this way has facilitated the study and treatment of hyperlipoproteinaemias but it is important to remember that each type is not necessarily a single disease entity and may have a number of causes.

The molecular defect that gives rise to a particular hyperlipoproteinaemia is known for some, but not all, of these diseases. Three examples of monogenic disorders of plasma lipoproteins will be described below. In some cases the molecular defect of two different genes can give rise to a similar phenotype. For example both a defect of the enzyme **lipoprotein lipase (LPL)** and of the protein **apoCII**, which is required to activate LPL, give rise to hyperchylomicronaemia which is characteristic of type I hyperlipoproteinaemia.

Some of the hyperlipoproteinaemias may be polygenic i.e. have defects of two or more genes, although this has not yet been clearly established. It is also important to remember that some of the hyperlipoproteinaemias are produced as secondary symptoms to other major clinical syndromes e.g. hypothyroidism and diabetes (see chapter 10).

The **European Atherosclerosis Society** have recommended some guidelines for recognising and treating patients with hyperlipoproteinaemia which will be discussed with the various methods of treatment available.

Table 5.1 Hyperlipoproteinaemias Cholesterol (C) Triacylglycerol (TAG)

Fredrickson Type *WHO phenotype*	*lipoprotein pattern* *plasma lipid concentration (mM)*	*main clinical features*	*molecular defect (if known)* *disease*
Type I	raised chylomicrons C<6.5 TAG 10-30	eruptive xanthomas lipaemia retinalis hepatosplenomegaly pancreatitis	LPL Familial Lipoprotein Lipase Deficiency or ApoCII
Type IIa	raised LDL C 7.5-16 TAG<2.3	premature coronary heart disease xanthomas corneal arcus	LDL receptor Familial Hypercholesterolaemia
Type IIb	raised LDL and VLDL C6.5-10 TAG 2.3-12	premature coronary heart disease xanthomas corneal arcus	
Type III	ß-VLDL C 9-14 TAG9-14	extensive vascular disease palmar xanthomas tuberoeruptive xanthomas	ApoE Dyslipoproteinaemia
Type IV	raised VLDL C 6.5-12 TAG 10-30	eruptive xanthomas lipaemia retinalis hepatosplenomegaly	
Type V	raised chylomicrons and VLDL C 6.5-12 TAG 10-30	eruptive xanthomas lipaemia retinalis hepatosplenomegaly	

5.2 Familial lipoprotein lipase deficiency (Fredrickson Type I)

Clinical symptoms and biochemical features

Many of the patients with this disease present with abdominal pain (about 60%) and some of these will have acute pancreatitis, which, if treatment is not effective, can prove fatal. The disease may become apparent in early childhood. There is often hepatosplenomegaly (enlarged liver and spleen) and frequently eruptive **xanthomas** (lipid depositions under the skin) are seen. These are localised on buttocks, knees and elbows and contain triacylglycerol enriched lipid laden cells. In about 20% of cases lipaemia retinalis is observed: the arterioles and venules of the retina assume a pale pink colour as the blood is loaded with the large lipoprotein particles, the chylomicrons.

A simple test, to demonstrate the accumulation of chylomicrons in a patient with this disorder, is to obtain a sample of the patient's plasma and leave it overnight at 4°C, after which a milky layer will develop at the top of the plasma.

It is interesting to note that Familial Lipoprotein Lipase deficiency is not usually accompanied by atherosclerosis. This is probably because chylomicrons are too large to enter the artery wall.

Molecular defect

The molecular defect is in the enzyme lipoprotein lipase. As described in chapter 4, this is the enzyme which hydrolyses triacylglycerol in chylomicrons and VLDL. It is synthesised in adipose cells, secreted into the bloodstream and is active, as a homodimer, when bound, via heparin sulphate to the surface of endothelial cells. The human gene for this enzyme is on chromosome 8, contains 10 exons and codes for a mature protein of 448 amino acids.

Numerous mutations of the LPL gene have been described, some of which are associated with reduced or inactive enzyme and hence with hyperchylomicronaemia. The clinical diagnosis of the disease requires a demonstration of reduced LPL activity and if possible identification of the defect in the LPL gene.

Familial Lipoprotein Lipase deficiency is just one of the hyperlipoproteinaemias that belong to the type I hyperlipoproteinaemia. A similar lipoprotein profile will occur if there is a defect of the apoCII gene.

Treatment

The main treatment is dietary fat restriction, thus limiting the formation of chylomicrons. Medium chain fatty acids may be included in the diet as these are absorbed directly into the portal vein without being incorporated into chylomicrons, but long chain fatty acids should be avoided.

5.3 Familial hypercholesterolaemia (Fredrickson Type IIa)

Patients with this disease suffer from premature coronary heart disease. The inheritance of this genetic disorder is by an autosomal dominant trait. Heterozygotes occur with a frequency of 1 in 500 whereas the homozygotes occur at 1 in 1,000,000.

Clinical symptoms and biochemical features

Xanthomas due to deposition of cholesterol, derived from LDL, occur in tendons and skin. In the heterozygotes, xanthomas develop by about 20 years and atherosclerosis by about 30 years, whereas in the homozygotes, the disease is more severe and begins earlier: death may occur from coronary heart disease by 20 years of age.

The WHO phenotype of this disease is type IIa. There is a dramatic increase in the amount of LDL found in the blood. In heterozygotes, the plasma cholesterol is increased by approximately two-fold but in the homozygote levels may be four to five times higher than normal.

Molecular defect

This disease is caused by a mutation of the gene for the low-density lipoprotein receptor (LDLr). This receptor enables the LDL particle to be taken up by cells by receptor mediated endocytosis as described in chapter 4. The receptor is normally expressed on most tissue cells. When the receptor is deficient, either in amount or in function, LDL accumulates in blood and is taken up, after modification, by the monocyte scavenger receptor. It is the accumulation of cholesterol in monocyte derived macrophages in skin and tendons that leads to formation of xanthomas and atherosclerosis in the arterial intima.

The LDLr gene is on the short arm of chromosome 19, in man, and comprises 18 exons. The gene codes for a single chain protein containing 839 amino acids in the mature protein. The structure of the receptor protein is described in chapter 4. More than 400 different mutations of the LDLr gene have been identified. On the basis of the behaviour of the mutant protein five groups of mutations have been identified:

1) Those which fail to produce immunoprecipitable protein
2) Those which give proteins which are not transported from the endoplasmic reticulum to the golgi
3) Those proteins which are transported to the plasma membrane but fail to bind LDL
4) Those proteins which do bind LDL but which are not internalised
5) Those proteins that transport LDL into the cell but which are unable to release the LDL into the lumen of the lysosome.

While the defect of the LDLr gene is primarily responsible for the increase plasma concentrations of LDL, the severity of the hypercholesterolaemia and the time of onset of the clinical symptoms of coronary heart disease is variable and may be affected by other factors.

Animal models of Familial Hypercholesterolaemia

The Watanabe Heritable Hyperlipidaemic rabbit is an animal model of this disease which has been much studied: the mutant LDL receptor in this strain of rabbit causes a very high plasma LDL concentration and a high incidence of severe coronary and aortic atherosclerosis. A transgenic mouse model of Familial Hypercholesterolaemia has been obtained by specific targeted destruction of the LDLr gene.

Treatment of Familial Hypercholesterolaemia

Only palliative treatment, such as a liver transplant as an extreme measure, is possible in the homozygote. However, gene therapy has been tried with limited success.

In the heterozygote measures to reduce plasma cholesterol by diet and drug treatment (discussed in more detail below) may reduce the severity of the symptoms and prolong life.

5.4 Dysbetalipoproteinaemia (Fredrickson Type III)

Clinical symptoms and biochemical features

This disease has a high incidence of coronary and peripheral atherosclerosis. Almost half the patients with this disorder also have a characteristic symptom: palmar xanthomas i.e. raised lipid filled lesions in the creases of the palms of the hand.

The disease has a recessive mode of inheritance and is rarely seen until early adulthood. It occurs more in men than women although it does occur in women after the menopause suggesting that oestrogen has a protective effect, preventing the appearance of clinical symptoms.

Both plasma cholesterol and triacylglycerol are elevated. The lipoprotein profile is characterised by an unusual lipoprotein, termed **ßVLDL** which is in fact cholesterol enriched very low-density lipoprotein and chylomicron remnants. The presence of these unusual lipoprotein particles gives rise to the other name for the disease: remnant particle disease.

Molecular defect

The defect is in the apoE gene. The apoE found in this disease is apoE2 which binds poorly to lipoprotein receptors thus disturbing lipoprotein metabolism and leading to progressive development of atherosclerosis and clinical symptoms. In the ApoE2 protein the amino acid arginine at position 158, seen in apoE3, is replaced by cysteine. The third form of apoE, apoE4 differs from apoE2 and apoE3 having an arginine residue at position 112 instead of cysteine. These three common alleles, ε2,ε3 and ε4, of the single structural gene locus can give rise to the homozygote E4/4, E3/3 and E2/2 and the heterozygote E4/3, E3/2 and E4/2 phenotypes. In patients with dysbetalipoproteinaemia over 90% have the E2/2 genotype. However, development of the clinical symptoms of dysbetalipoproteinaemia, in individuals with this genotype, requires some additional precipitating condition such as hypothyroidism, obesity or diabetes to be present. This is clearly obvious from the fact that while 1:100 people are E2/E2 homozygous less than 1:5,000 develop dysbetalipoproteinaemia.

The majority of the apoE found in blood is synthesised by the liver but is also produced by other tissues. The apoE gene, which is on chromosome 19, in man, contains 4 exons and codes for a primary translation product of 317 amino acids. The 18 amino terminal amino acids act as a signal peptide and are absent from the secreted mature protein. Before secretion the apoE is modified by glycosylation: a carbohydrate chain containing sialic acid residues, is added to the protein on threonine 194. The sialic acid residues are subsequently partially removed in the plasma, contributing to the apparent polymorphism of plasma apoE.

The accumulation of remnant particles is probably due to reduced binding of the mutant apoE to the LDL receptor and also possibly to heparin sulphate proteoglycans and to the LRP receptor on the surface of hepatic cells. Thus the removal of these particles from the circulation is impaired.

Animal model of dysbetalipoproteinaemia

A transgenic rabbit has been described which expresses apoE2 and has the symptoms of dysbetalipoproteinaemia. Several different transgenic mice models have been obtained to investigate the role of apoE in lipoprotein metabolism and atherosclerosis.

Treatment of dysbetalipoproteinaemia

Control of dietary intake, with restricted fat content, is the first method of treatment. Drug treatment may also be necessary. **Nicotinic acid**, fibric acid derivatives or **HMGCoA reductase inhibitors**, all of which are described below, are effective in lowering plasma lipid levels and reducing the risk of myocardial infarct, angina and intermittent claudication, the clinical symptoms which are seen in this disease when untreated.

5.5 Other hyperlipoproteinaemias

The above three hyperlipoproteinaemias are caused by specific molecular defects in certain proteins produced by gene mutations that have been identified. Another specific gene mutation that produces symptoms that are indistinguishable from familial hypercholesterolaemia is the substitution of glutamine for arginine at position 3,500 of apoB. This dominantly inherited disorder results in a protein with reduced affinity for the LDL receptor.

The hyperlipoproteinaemia known as **familial combined hyperlipoproteinaemia** is a clinical entity but this may represent a heterogeneous group of genetic defects that have not yet been fully elucidated. The common biochemical feature of familial combined hyperlipoproteinaemia is an overproduction of apoB containing lipoproteins by the liver i.e. an overproduction of VLDL. The resulting phenotype will depend upon the subsequent catabolism of VLDL. Although this disease does not usually become evident until the late teens or early twenties it requires prompt treatment as these patients are at a high risk of developing coronary heart disease.

Several of the WHO phenotypes are found as secondary symptoms of other major diseases such as hypothyroidism, nephrotic syndrome, liver disease such as primary biliary cirrhosis, diabetes and obesity. Corticosteroid hormones and certain drugs may also alter the lipoprotein profile adversely and produce a hyperlipoproteinaemia. The secondary hyperlipoproteinaemias associated with obesity and diabetes will be discussed further in chapter 10.

5.6 Hyperlipoproteinaemia and atherosclerosis

As mentioned above, it is significant that Familial Lipoprotein Lipase deficiency is not usually accompanied by atherosclerosis: the chylomicrons that accumulate in the blood are thought to be too large to enter the artery wall. However, when LDL accumulates in blood, as in Familial Hypercholesterolaemia and other hypercholesterolaemias, extensive atherosclerosis develops and premature cardiovascular disease occurs.

Severe cardiovascular disease also accompanies dysbetalipoproteinaemia. In this disorder the lipoproteins which accumulates in the blood are cholesterol enriched VLDL remnants. These particles may not be dissimilar in size to LDL but they differ from the latter due to the presence of apoE. The evidence suggests that they too can cause atherogenesis. It is also possible that the VLDL receptor may have a role in the development of atherosclerosis. The VLDL receptor has been shown to be present on the endothelium of capillaries and small arterioles and in atherosclerotic lesions.

5.7 Treatment of hyperlipoproteinaemias

The European Atherosclerosis Society has recommended some guidelines for the treatment of patients with elevated plasma lipid levels. These recommendations are shown in table 2.

Table 5.2 Treatment of hyperlipidaemias recommended by the European Atherosclerosis Society

Group	*Description*	*Plasma cholesterol (mM)*	*Plasma TAG (mM)*	*Relative risk of coronary heart disease*	*Treatment*
A	slightly elevated cholesterol, low TAG	5.2-6.5	<2.3	two fold at 6.5mM cholesterol	Diet: reduce fat
B	moderately elevated cholesterol, low TAG	6.5-7.8	<2.3	four fold at 7.8mM cholesterol	Diet: reduce fat Drug therapy
C	low cholesterol, moderately elevated TAG	<5.2	2.3-5.6	Hypertri-glyceridaemia may be associated with other risk factors such as obesity and diabetes	Treat other risk factors Diet: reduce fat and calories if weight reduction necessary
D	elevated cholesterol, moderately elevated TAG	5.2-7.8	2.3-5.6	high risk	Diet and drug therapy
E	high cholesterol, high TAG	>7.8	5.6	extremely high risk	Diet and drug therapy essential

The general practitioner will try to establish from the patient's medical history whether the high plasma lipids are secondary to some other underlying disease, such as hypothyroidism or diabetes, which must be treated first, or whether there is a primary hyperlipidaemia associated with a genetic defect. He will also take into account the presence of other risk factors such as obesity, hypertension and smoking. Counselling to remove or reduce these risk factors should accompany dietary or drug treatment of the hyperlipidaemia and the patient must have regular medical follow up to assess the effectiveness of treatment.

Diet

The first method of treatment of hyperlipidaemia is to modify the diet so that, if necessary, weight loss occurs and the fat content, particularly the saturated fat, is reduced. The effect of dietary fat upon plasma lipid levels is discussed in detail in chapter 7. It is often possible to lower total plasma cholesterol and LDL cholesterol by suitable adjustments to the diet.

However, when the hyperlipidaemia is severe, dietary measures may not be sufficient to lower the plasma levels to those which are deemed less of a risk for developing coronary heart disease and other cardiovascular problems. A prudent diet should then be accompanied by some form of drug therapy. The major types of drugs used for lipid lowering are described below.

Bile acid sequestrant resins

Resins, such as cholestyramine, may be administered as a powder, dispersed in fruit juice. Cholestyramine is a large molecular weight polystyrene polymer with divinylbenzene cross-links and quarternary ammonium groups. The resins are not absorbed and act to prevent re-absorption of bile acids. This increases cholesterol secretion from the liver and increases LDL receptor activity in the liver. Plasma LDL cholesterol may be lowered 20-30% by regular consumption of about 20g of resin per day.

Some side effects may be observed in some patients and care must be taken to supplement the diet with certain vitamins whose absorption is reduced by the resins. Their use also tends to stimulate hepatic cholesterol synthesis that partially offsets the benefit of increased cholesterol excretion. These drugs are most often used to treat heterozygote familial hypercholesterolaemia and are increasingly used in combination with cholesterol synthesis inhibitors which prevent the stimulation of hepatic cholesterol synthesis (see below).

Fibrates

These drugs, which include clofibrate and gemfibrozil (see figure 5.1.) have a number of biochemical effects: they decrease VLDL production and increase VLDL catabolism by increasing the activity of LPL. The level of plasma LDL cholesterol may be decreased although this effect is variable.

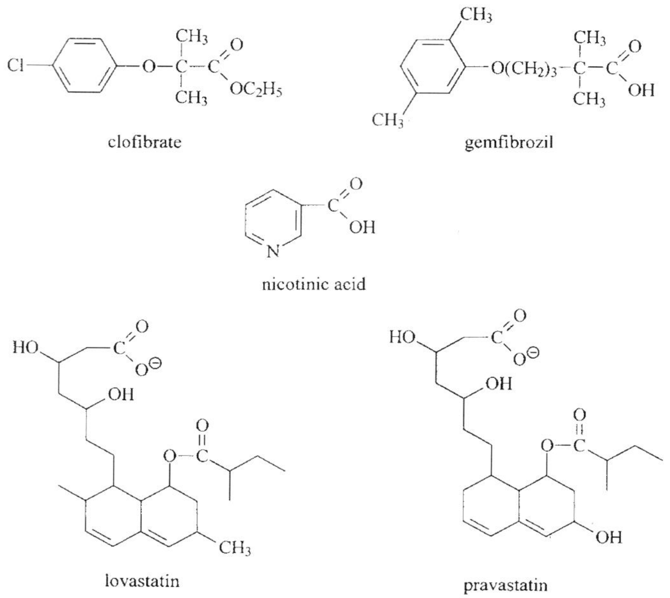

Figure 5.1
Some lipid lowering drugs

Some side effects are observed in some patients such as increased incidence of cholesterol gallstones.

These drugs belong to a class of compounds known as peroxisomal proliferators and may act through the regulation of gene expression by modulation of the activity of nuclear receptors termed **peroxisomal proliferator activated receptor -alpha (PPARα)**.

Nicotinic acid

When used in pharmacological doses nicotinic acid (see figure 5.1.) reduces VLDL and LDL production and hence can be a valuable lipid lowering drug.

Side effects of flushing can be avoided by taking aspirin shortly before the nicotinic acid dose.

Cholesterol synthesis inhibitors

The inhibitors of HMGCoA reductase are potent cholesterol lowering drugs. These include lovastatin and pravastatin (see figure 5.1.). Large reductions in LDL cholesterol can be achieved at comparatively low doses of drug, which are well tolerated.

Lovastatin and pravastatin have been tested (separately) in five year long trials and continue to be effective after this time period without adverse effects. Lovastatin produced a small increase in HDL cholesterol and was equally effective in the reduction of LDL cholesterol in heterozygous familial hypercholesterolaemia, non-familial hypercholesterolaemia and combined hyperlipoproteinaemia. The trial of pravastatin was carried out in hypercholesterolaemic men who at the beginning of the trial did not have a history of myocardial infarction. It was found that treatment with the cholesterol synthesis inhibitor significantly lowered LDL cholesterol (by 26%) and reduced the incidence of myocardial infarction and death from cardiovascular causes (see chapter 2). The emergence of these highly effective drugs, with little evidence of side effects, have made them the treatment of choice for hypercholesterolaemia.

LDL apheresis

Removal of LDL from blood, extracorporeally, is termed **LDL apheresis**. This procedure which is analogous to kidney dialysis is usually performed once a fortnight and is successful in reducing LDL levels. It should be reserved for patients whose lipoprotein profile is refractory to drug treatment, such as those suffering from homozygous familial hypercholesterolaemia. However, long-term studies, in which this treatment has been used for five years show that it is relatively safe and effective in reducing cardiovascular incidences.

Gene therapy

The possibility of replacing an abnormal LDLr gene with a normal gene has been investigated. Removal of a portion of liver, transfection of the liver cells with a recombinant retrovirus containing a normal human LDLr gene and transfer of these cells back to the patient *via* a portal venous catheter has been successfully achieved. However, the modest cholesterol-lowering achieved, set against the risk involved in such surgery, mean that further investigation is required before considering routine use of such a technique.

A potential gene therapy method for the treatment of dysbetalipoproteinaemia in man is to enable the liver to express the VLDL receptor by transfection of the VLDLr gene. This has been described to reduce hypercholesterolaemia in apoE2 transgenic mice.

5.8 Conclusion

The study of the hyperlipoproteinaemias has improved the understanding of lipoprotein metabolism and of the development of atherosclerosis. As several of the hyperlipoproteinaemias are accompanied by premature cardiovascular disease the successful treatment of the hyperlipidaemia will reduce the incidence of clinical events such as angina, myocardial infarct and stroke.

The main aim of treatment of the hyperlipoproteinaemias is to reduce plasma lipid concentrations. However, the treatment of underlying diseases such as hypothyroidism, diabetes and obesity is necessary in the secondary hyperlipoproteinaemias. For primary hyperlipoproteinaemias the initial treatment is to improve the diet. If dietary intervention is not effective then various drugs are available. A combination of drug treatments may be more effective in lowering plasma cholesterol. LDL apheresis and gene therapy are more extreme forms of treatment for certain hyperlipoproteinaemias. These may be confined to monogenic homozygous disorders where the prognosis is very poor.

We have concentrated on the well-known risk factor for coronary heart disease-elevated cholesterol levels in plasma, particularly in LDL. However, many high-risk patients also have elevated plasma TAG levels and the role of plasma TAG, as a risk factor remains controversial and subject for debate.

According to Grundy (1998), "Current evidence indicates that hypercholesterolaemia directly causes atherosclerosis whereas hypertriglyceridaemia is better viewed as a marker for increased coronary artery disease risk."

Key references

General references

Scriver, C.R., Beaudet, A.L., Sly, W.S. and Valle, D. (1995) The metabolic and molecular bases of inherited diseases, vol II seventh edition McGraw-Hill Inc.

Stein, E.A. and MyersLipids, G.L. (1994) Lipoproteins and apolipoproteins. In: Tietz Textbook of Clinical Chemistry (ed C.A. Burts, E.R. Ashwood). W.B. Saunders Co, second edition. 1002-1093

Tietz textbook of Clinical Chemistry (1994) ed. C.A.Burtis and E.R.Ashwood pub. W.B.Saunders Co, second edition.

Familial lipoprotein lipase deficiency

Goldberg, I.J. (1996) Lipoprotein lipase and lipolysis: central role in lipoprotein metabolism. Journal of Lipid Research 37, 693-707

Familial Hypercholesterolaemia

Rosenfeld, M.E., Tsukada, T., Gown, A.M. and Ross, R. (1987) Fatty streak initiation in Watanabe Heritable Hyperlipidaemic and comparably hypercholesterolaemic fat-fed rabbits. Arteriosclerosis 7, 9-23

Ishibashi, S., Goldstein, J.L., Brown, M.S., Herz, J. and Burns, D.K. (1994) Massive xanthomatosis and atherosclerosis in cholesterol fed low density lipoprotein receptor negative mice. Journal of Clinical Investigation 93, 1885-1893

Sun, X.M. *et al.* (1998) Influence of genotype at the low density lipoprotein (LDL) receptor gene locus on the clinical phenotype and response to lipid lowering drug therapy in heterozygous familial hypercholesterolaemia. Atherosclerosis 136, 175-185

Dysbetalipoproteinaemia

Zannis, V.I. (1986) Genetic polymorphism in Human Apolipoprotein E. Methods in Enzymology 128, 823-851

Dallongville, J., Lussier-Cacan, S. and Davignon, J. (1992) Modulation of plasma triglyceride levels by apo E phenotype: a meta analysis. Journal of Lipid Research 33, 447-454

Huang, Y. *et al.* (1997) Apolipoprotein E2 transgenic rabbits. Modulation of type III hyperlipoproteinaemia phenotype by oestrogen and occurrence of spontaneous atherosclerosis. Journal of Biological Chemistry 272, 22685-22694

Hofker, M.H., Van Vlijonen, B.J.M. and Haveker, L.M. (1998) Transgenic mouse models to study the role of apoE in hyperlipidemia and atherosclerosis. Atherosclerosis 137, 1-11

Other hyperlipoproteinaemias

Wang, X.L., McCredie, R.M. and Wilcken, D.E.L. (1995) Polymorphisms of the apolipoprotein E gene and severity of coronary artery disease defined by angiography. Arterosclerosis, Thrombosis and Vascular Biolology 15, 1030-1034

Myant, N.B. (1993) Familial defective apolipoprotein B-100: a review, including some comparisons with familial hypercholesterolaemia. Atherosclerosis 104, 1-18

Treatment of hyperlipoproteinaemias

Study Group, European Atherosclerosis Society. (1988) The recognition and management of hyperlipidaemia in adults: A policy statement of the European Atherosclerosis Society. European Heart Journal 9, 571-600

Cholesterol synthesis inhibitors

Tikkanen, M.J., Ojala, J. and Helve, E. (1992) Long term use of lovastatin in different types of hyperlipaemia. Atherosclerosis 97 S27-S32

Shepherd, J. *et al.* (1995) Prevention of coronary heart disease with pravastatin in men with hypercholesterolaemia. New England Journal of Medicine 333, 1301-1307

LDL apheresis

Gorden, B.R. *et al.* (1998) Long term effects of low density lipoprotein apheresis using an automated dextran sulfate cellulose adsorption system. American Journal of Cardiology 81, 407-411

Gene therapy

Raper, S.E. *et al.* (1996) Safety and feasibility of liver directed ex vivo gene replacement therapy for homozygous familial hypercholesterolaemia. Annals of Surgery 223, 116-126

Van Dijk, K.W. *et al.* (1998) Reversal of hypercholesterolaemia in apolipoprotein E2 and apolipoprotein E3-Leiden transgenic mice by adenovirus mediated gene transfer of the VLDL receptor. Arteriosclerosis, Thrombosis and Vascular Biology 18, 7-12

Conclusion

Grundy, S.M. (1998) Hypertriglyceridemia, atherogenic dyslipidemia and the metabolic syndrome (1998) American Journal of Cardiology 81 (4A), 18B-25B

6 Lipoproteins and Atherosclerosis

6.1 Introduction

One of the major risk factors for the development of atherosclerotic disease is an elevated plasma cholesterol, particularly the cholesterol of the lipoprotein, LDL. Risk factors are discussed in chapter 3 and the properties of lipoproteins are discussed in chapter 4. The role played by LDL and other lipoproteins in the development and progression of atherosclerosis will be considered in detail below. Epidemiological studies suggest a strong correlation between plasma LDL concentration and the incidence of atherosclerotic disease but such investigations do not answer the following vital question: does elevated LDL cause atherosclerosis or does it aggravate the disease, already present?

There is good evidence supporting a major role of increased LDL in the initiation of atherosclerotic lesion formation and also in the progression of lesions to more advanced forms, although other factors may be involved, particularly in the latter stages of the disease process.

Atherosclerosis is a disease of the intima so, to understand the disease process in biochemical terms, it is necessary to consider the biochemistry of the normal intima. The normal integration of metabolism and maintenance of homeostasis is disrupted in atherosclerosis. The various ways in which intimal biochemistry is altered in atherosclerosis will be discussed so that some insight into the mechanism(s) of disease initiation, development and progression can be obtained.

6.2 LDL and atheroma formation

Transendothelial transport of LDL

Although the endothelial cells form a barrier between blood and the underlying intimal layer, lipoproteins are present in the intima and their concentration in the intima reflects the plasma concentration. LDL can enter endothelial cells by endocytosis either by a LDL receptor mediated mechanism or a receptor independent process *via* plasmalemmal vesicles (vesicles of plasma membrane). Both mechanisms can transport LDL to lysosomes to supply endothelial cells with cholesterol. Endothelial cells can also transport LDL across the endothelium to the underlying intima *via* plasmalemmal vesicles, a process termed **transcytosis**.

Studies have been made, *in vitro*, using a monolayer of human umbilical endothelial cells grown on a porous filter, of trans-endothelial transport of LDL. LDL was transported across the endothelial cell layer by a receptor-independent route and the rate of transport was concentration dependent. Some receptor-dependent uptake occurred which led to lipoprotein degradation within the endothelial cell. Interestingly, the rate of transport from the lower to the upper surface of the endothelial layer (equivalent to transport from the intima to the lumen of the artery), was several fold higher than transport in the other direction. Such asymmetric transport, if it occurs *in vivo*, would tend to oppose accumulation of macromolecules in the intima. Thus, other processes must be operative *in vivo* to permit the accumulation of lipid in the intima which is seen in atherosclerosis.

It has been shown, using porcine aortic cells in culture, that high LDL concentrations alter the permeability of endothelial cells to macromolecules, including LDL. This was accompanied by a selective decrease in the basement membrane associated heparin sulphate proteoglycan. If these effects occur, *in vivo*, then high concentrations of LDL in the blood may have a role in the initiation of atherosclerosis by altering the permeability of the endothelium and promoting endothelial dysfunction.

In cholesterol-fed rabbits the LDL concentration in the artery wall is almost six fold higher in the sites susceptible to developing atherosclerotic lesions, known as **lesion prone sites**, compared with the concentration in lesion-resistant sites. Thus the concentration of lipoprotein in the intima is not necessarily uniform throughout the vasculature. The focal accumulation of LDL may be a prerequisite for lesion formation. Lesion-prone sites are also observed in the human arterial system (see chapter 2).

Factors such as high blood pressure, smoking, genetic factors, infection and small sized LDL may increase endothelial permeability to LDL. Thus, when the plasma lipoprotein concentrations are elevated, an increased permeability to lipoproteins may be a further factor in the development of atherosclerosis in humans.

The interaction of LDL with the extracellular matrix proteoglycans also has an important part to play in the development and progression of atherosclerosis. The smaller sized LDL particles have more of the apoB present on the surface of the lipoprotein particle in an orientation that binds to extracellular proteoglycans than larger lipoprotein particles. A specific sequence of positively charged amino acids in the apoB, within the LDL receptor-binding region, has a high affinity for the negatively charged sulphate and carboxyl residues in the glycosaminoglycan chains of the proteoglycans. This interaction could remove the LDL from the fluid pool of the intima thus providing a concentration gradient to allow more LDL to enter the intima. The binding of LDL to matrix proteoglycans may also increase the residence time of the LDL particles in the intima thus increasing the opportunity for the LDL to undergo modification as described below.

Monocyte adhesion and transmigration

As explained in chapter 2 the arterial intima normally contains few macrophages. However in atherosclerosis, macrophages accumulate in the intima and are derived from circulating monocytes which first adhere to the arterial endothelial cells and then penetrate the sub-endothelial space. It has not been fully established what promotes monocyte adhesion and transmigration across the endothelium *in vivo*. However, in cells in culture, the adhesivity of monocytes to endothelial cells is enhanced by pre-incubation of monocytes with LDL. LDL appears to stimulate the production of **monocyte chemotactic protein** that promotes transmigration of human monocytes into the sub-endothelial space. Thus, LDL may play a role in the initial events that lead to the development of fatty streaks by promoting monocyte adhesion and transmigration.

Cell contact between endothelial cells and monocytes induces further synthesis of monocyte chemotactic protein in both types of cells. Monocyte chemotactic protein secretion, by endothelial cells, is also increased by mechanical stress. Monocyte chemotactic protein is also produced by sub-intimal monocytes and this may be important in subsequent recruitment of further monocytes.

The expression of the adhesion molecules, **P-selectin** and **vascular cell adhesion molecule-1 (VCAM-1)** precedes the appearance of macrophages in the artery wall and lesion development. Hence the synthesis of specific adhesion molecules, by endothelial cells, is an early event in atherogenesis.

Foam cell formation: LDL modification, LDL oxidation and the scavenger receptor

In atherosclerotic lesions macrophages become filled with lipid droplets. These cells acquire a spongy appearance: hence the term **foam cells**. The major lipid that accumulates is cholesterol ester from LDL. Macrophages, *in vitro*, cannot be converted to foam cells in the presence of native LDL but can accumulate lipid from **modified LDL** *via* the **scavenger receptor** (see chapter 4) and become foam cells. LDL can be modified, *in vitro*, to a form recognised by the scavenger receptor, by incubating LDL with cultured endothelial cells, macrophages or metal ions such as copper or iron. The modification that produces **oxidised LDL**, is the result of peroxidation of polyunsaturated fatty acids of surface phospholipids in the LDL particle. Formation of lipid peroxides is followed by fragmentation of fatty acids to short chain aldehydes such as malondialdehyde and 4-hydroxynonenal that bind to apoB and thus alter the binding specificity of the LDL molecule. Some oxidation of cholesterol, within LDL, also occurs. Oxidation of LDL is discussed further in chapter 9.

Oxidised LDL has been detected in atherosclerotic lesions of the rabbit and humans. Detailed analysis of the distribution of LDL and oxidised LDL in atherosclerotic lesions of rabbits shows that the latter are mainly cell associated in macrophage rich fatty streaks whereas native LDL has a limited diffuse distribution and was mainly extracellular. In more advanced atheroma native and oxidised LDL are trapped in the extracellular matrix. The intracellular accumulation of oxidised LDL in macrophages is in part due to the resistance of the modified apoB to degradation by lysosomal enzymes.

The oxidation of LDL, as described above, can be induced *in vitro* by a variety of cells including endothelial cell and macrophages. Oxidative modification of LDL by endothelial cells may occur through the activity of a 15-lipoxygenase. The extracellular oxidation of LDL by macrophages, that may occur by release of oxidised unsaturated fatty acids from these cells, is dependent upon the LDL binding to the LDL receptor on the macrophage. Once oxidised the modified LDL then becomes a ligand for the scavenger receptor and is internalised by the macrophage. LDL can also be modified, *in vitro*, by peroxynitrite, a reactive oxygen species discussed below, to a form recognised by the scavenger receptor.

Minimally modified LDL, in which there is only limited peroxidation of fatty acids and no significant alteration of the charge on apoB, stimulates the release from endothelial cells of the monocyte chemotactic protein. Further oxidation of LDL produces a form that is taken up by macrophages by the scavenger receptor. Oxidised LDL stimulates a number of biochemical reactions, some of which have been observed *in vivo* and some in tissue culture systems (table 6.1).

Other modifications of LDL may also occur within the intima. For example, the enzyme *phospholipase A2*, which is secreted by macrophages and endothelial cells, can act upon phosphatidylcholine in the LDL surface and produce lysophosphatidylcholine (lysolecithin). The latter molecule has been shown in cell culture experiments to stimulate smooth muscle cell proliferation. If this occurred, *in vivo*, in the intima it would contribute to the progression of atherosclerosis. Another enzyme, which has been observed to occur in higher concentrations in the extracellular matrix in atherosclerotic lesions than in the normal artery wall, which could modify LDL, is *sphingomyelinase*.

Table 6.1
Effect of oxidised LDL on cells of the arterial intima (adapted from Holvoet and Collen, 1994).

Effect of oxLDL to promote:	*Projected consequence in vivo*
Endothelial cells	
Synthesis of adhesion molecules	Adhesion of monocytes
Synthesis of monocyte chemotactic protein	Transmigration of monocytes from lumen to intima
Synthesis of macrophage colony stimulating factor	Proliferation of monocytes and macrophages
Synthesis of growth factors	Proliferation of smooth muscle cells and growth of neointima
Reduced secretion of nitric oxide: half life of mRNA for nitric oxide synthase reduced from 36h to 10h	Vasoconstriction and platelet aggregation
Increased secretion of endothelin	Vasoconstriction
Secretion of prostaglandins	Platelet aggregation
Reduced synthesis of protein C and enhanced synthesis of Tissue Factor	Thrombin generation, platelet aggregation and coagulation
Reduced synthesis of plasminogen activator and stimulation of synthesis of plasminogen activator inhibitor	Defective fibrinolysis
Monocyte/macrophages	
Synthesis of monocyte chemotactic protein	Chemoattraction of monocytes
Uptake of oxidised LDL	Formation of foam cells
Increased antigen presenting capacity	Activation of the immune response
Smooth muscle cells	
Chemoattraction	Migration of smooth muscle cells and growth of neointima
Synthesis of platelet-derived growth factor	Migration of smooth muscle cells
Synthesis of basic fibroblast growth factor	Proliferation of smooth muscle cells

This enzyme hydrolyses sphingomyelin in the surface of LDL to ceramide and phosphocholine. The action of sphingomyelinase on LDL induces aggregation and fusion of LDL particles which increases the affinity of LDL for proteoglycans. Oxidation of LDL, in contrast, decreases the affinity of the lipoprotein for proteoglycans.

The presence of oxidised LDL in atherosclerotic lesions and the anti-atherogenic effect of antioxidants (see chapter 9) supports a pathogenic role for oxidised LDL although the mechanism(s) of oxidation of LDL *in vivo* remains uncertain. Such a role is further supported by the biochemical effects of oxidised LDL all of which favour atherosclerosis (table 6.1). Some of the early events in atherogenesis are shown in figure 6.1 and summarised in figure 6.2.

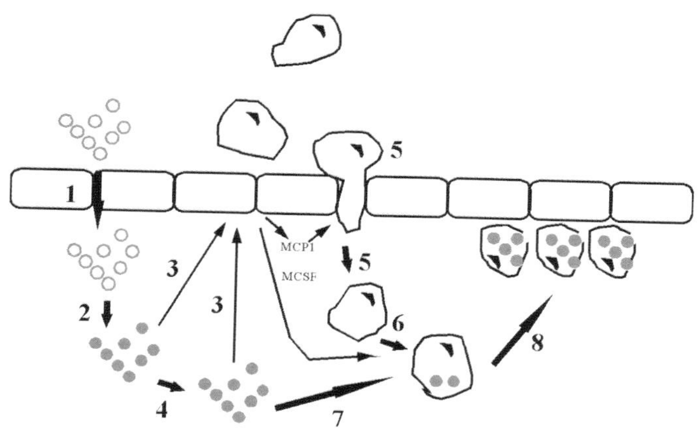

Figure 6.1 Early events of atherosclerosis (adapted from Berliner *et al*, 1995)

Abbreviations. mmLDL minimally modified LDL, oxLDL oxidised LDL, MCP1 monocyte chemotactic protein 1, MCSF macrophage colony stimulating factor.

Steps:
1. Transendothelial migration of LDL
2. Lipid oxidation
3. mmLDL and oxLDL stimulates MCP1 and MCSF secretion by endothelial cells
4. Further lipid oxidation
5. Adhesion and transmigration of monocytes
6. Differentiation of monocytes to macrophages
7. Uptake of oxLDL by macrophages
8. Formation of foam cells

6.3 HDL and atherogenesis

The observation that the incidence of coronary heart disease is inversely related to the concentration of HDL suggests that HDL has a protective effect, either preventing or slowing the development of atherosclerotic disease. This lipoprotein may protect against the development of atherosclerosis in two ways: by enhancing cholesterol efflux from the

Development	Influx of LDL Retention of LDL Oxidation of LDL Monocyte adhesion Monocyte migration Monocyte differentiation to macrophages Macrophage accumulation of oxLDL Foam cell formation
Progression	Further monocyte recruitment Macrophage proliferation Macrophage foam cell death and formation of lipid core Migration and proliferation of smooth muscle cells Formation of smooth muscle cell foam cells Formation of new extracellular matrix Fissure of lesion, thrombosis in artery lumen above lesion Incorporation of whole or part of thrombus into lesion Fibrosis of lesion Angiogenesis-formation of new blood vessels in lesion Calcification of some lesions

Figure 6.2
Events of development and progression of atherosclerosis

artery wall and by preventing the oxidation of lipids in LDL. Like LDL, the HDL particles can cross the endothelium into the intima and it is there that they exert their protective role.

Cholesterol efflux from the artery wall

The role of HDL and of its apolipoproteins in removing cholesterol from cells is discussed in chapter 4. In Tangiers disease there is a defect in the mechanism whereby apolipoproteins remove cholesterol and macrophage foam cells are manifest in tissues. In this disease plasma HDL levels are low, due to increased turnover, and LDL levels are also low. Despite the latter, some of these patients develop cardiovascular disease showing the importance of the removal of cholesterol in preventing the progression of atherosclerosis.

Antioxidant properties of HDL

A small proportion of HDL molecules contain the enzyme ***paraoxasone***. This enzyme destroys the phospholipids containing multioxygenated polyunsaturated fatty acids in oxidised LDL particles. If these are not destroyed by paraoxasone, they may fragment and become the substrates for a second enzyme found in HDL. This enzyme, ***platelet activating factor acetyl hydrolase***, hydrolyses damaged and potentially harmful phospholipids, in minimally modified LDL, to lysophospholipids and inactive fatty acid fragments. In plasma the activity of this enzyme is also associated with LDL.

6.4 Biochemistry of the normal intima

The biological functions of the cells and extracellular matrix of the arterial intima was outlined in chapter 2. The major biochemical functions of the intima, relevant to the development of atherosclerosis, will be discussed below.

Nitric oxide

The relaxation of blood vessels in response to acetylcholine is dependent on the release of **nitric oxide** from endothelial cells. The major stimulus of nitric oxide synthesis, *in vivo,* is believed to be increased shear stress (see below), which is exerted on the luminal surface of the endothelium by the flow of blood. Thus a decrease in the diameter of a vessel, at constant blood flow, will increase shear stress and stimulate nitric oxide secretion that stimulates smooth muscle relaxation to counteract the initial vasoconstriction. In addition, nitric oxide synthesis by endothelial cells may occur in response to decreased oxygen tension and, via membrane receptors, to acetylcholine and endothelin.

Nitric oxide synthase (L-arginine, NADPH:oxidoreductase, NO-forming, EC 1.14.13.39) catalyses the formation of citrulline and nitric oxide from arginine and NADPH. The reaction is complex, involving a five electron oxidation and requring oxygen, haem, FAD, FMN and tetrahydrobiopterin. The endothelial enzyme requires calcium and calmodulin for both of the reactions outlined below.

H_2N–C(=NH)–NH–R (O_2 → H_2O; NADPH → $NADP^+$) → H_2N–C(=N-OH)–NH–R (O_2 → H_2O; NADPH → $NADP^+$) → H_2N–C(=O)–NH–R + NO

arginine — hydroxyarginine — citrulline — nitric oxide

Endothelial nitric oxide synthase is constitutively expressed but can be induced by shear stress and by oestrogen. The enzyme is N-terminally myristoylated and is also palmitoylated. The former may facilitate binding to the golgi membrane while the latter facilitates binding to the caveolae in the plasma membrane. Activity of the enzyme may be regulated by phosphorylation which inactivates it and promotes dissociation from the membrane to the cytoplasm. In addition to endothelial nitric oxide synthase (eNOS) there are other isoforms of this enzyme: nNOS was first described in neuronal tissue and iNOS was originally described in macrophages.

Nitric oxide appears to have several functions in the normal intima. These include; a) promotion of smooth muscle relaxation, b) inhibition of platelet adherence and aggregation, c) action as an antioxidant and d) inhibition of smooth muscle proliferation. Nitric oxide stimulates muscle relaxation through the activation of *guanylate cyclase*. Nitric oxide stimulates this enzyme, both in endothelial cells and smooth muscle cells, by binding to the haem iron in the catalytic site, and increasing the synthesis of cGMP. The consequence of nitric oxide stimulation of cGMP formation in smooth muscle cells is a reduction in intracellular calcium available for contraction and hence relaxation occurs.

Nitric oxide, although it has an unpaired electron and is thus a paramagnetic, free radical species, is also an uncharged and fairly non-polar molecule which is able to freely diffuse through lipid membranes. Its solubility in water is similar to oxygen: 2-3mM. Although nitric oxide can react with oxygen in the gaseous phase to form nitrogen dioxide and in water to form NO_2^-, the reactions occur slowly at physiological concentrations and are probably not significant *in vivo*, under normal circumstances.

Nitric oxide can react with superoxide and this may represent a protective effect since superoxide can oxidise lipids. Superoxide radicals are normally efficiently removed by the enzyme *superoxide dismutase*. This enzyme has three isoforms: an extracellular enzyme, a cytoplasmic CuZn-enzyme and a mitochondrial matrix Mn-enzyme. As superoxide does not cross membranes very well, each enzyme functions to protect it's particular location. The extracellular enzyme is present in relatively high amounts in human intima. It is secreted by smooth muscle cells and is probably anchored in the extracellular matrix bound to heparin sulphate proteoglycan. This enzyme should protect extracellular lipoprotein, in transit across the intima, from being oxidised by superoxide anions.

Nitric oxide may exert further protective effects as an antioxidant, as it can rapidly react with organic hydroperoxy radicals and inhibit radical chain propagation: the peroxynitrolipids, once formed, rapidly decompose. Lipid peroxy radicals are intermediates in the oxidation of LDL (see chapter 9): thus nitric oxide could protect LDL from oxidation.

Nitric oxide synthesis may prevent the expression of monocyte chemotactic protein in the normal endothelium. In human umbilical vein endothelial cells in culture, the inhibition of nitric oxide synthesis was accompanied by an increase of monocyte chemotactic protein mRNA and active protein whereas the exogenous addition of nitric oxide gave a dose dependent decrease in mRNA and protein. A further potential protective effect of nitric oxide in the endothelium is the repression of macrophage colony stimulating factor gene expression.

Endothelin

Endothelial cells synthesise **endothelin-1**: other isoforms of this vasoconstrictor peptide are produced in other tissues. Endothelin-1 has 21 amino acid residues and two disulphide bridges. The latter are in the N-terminal region: in the C-terminal region are a group of hydrophobic amino acids that are involved in binding to the endothelin receptor. The structure of endothelin-1 has homology with the cardiotoxic peptides, the sarafotoxins, produced in the venom of the Israeli burrowing asp, *Atractaspis engaddensis*, and a similarity to the neurotoxins produced by scorpions. Although the physiological role of endothelin-1 has not been fully established it is believed to have a role in the regulation of vascular tone .

Endothelin-1 can contract vascular and nonvascular smooth muscle. The contraction is slow in onset and of a long duration. Intravenous injection of endothelin to experimental animals produces an initial rapid fall and then a sustained increase in blood pressure. However, *in vivo*, most of the endothelin secreted by the endothelium does not enter the blood stream but is secreted into the subendothelial intima and probably acts locally on the underlying smooth muscle cells. The EC_{50} for vasoconstrictive activity in porcine coronary arteries is $3x10^{-10}M$, which is a hundred fold more potent than angiotensin II.

The two main subtypes of endothelin receptor, ET_A and ET_B, which have been cloned and sequenced, appear to mediate contraction and relaxation respectively. The former receptors are found on smooth muscle cells and the latter on endothelial cells. When endothelin binds to ET_A a *phospholipase C* is activated and inositol 1,4,5-triphosphate and diacylglycerol are produced. These second messengers stimulate the release of stored Ca^{2+} from the sarcoplasmic reticulum and the activation of protein kinase C respectively. Endothelin-1 also stimulates the entry of extracellular Ca^{2+} and the subsequent increased intracellular Ca^{2+} facilitates muscle contraction in smooth muscle cells. In endothelial cells a *phospholipase D* and *phospholipase A* may be activated, the former producing phosphatidic acid and the latter indirectly producing prostaglandins.

Shear stress

The main stimulus of the change of arterial diameter *in vivo* is a cha, of shear stress. Several biochemical changes induced by changes i, shear stress have been described in endothelial cells in culture. These biochemical changes may occur rapidly, within minutes, or may take some hours to take effect.

The forces acting on the artery wall can be resolved into two vectors, one perpendicular to the artery wall which is the blood pressure and one parallel to the wall which is the shear force. The latter can be considered as a frictional force produced by blood flowing over the endothelial surface. As blood flow is pulsatile, shear stress will continually be changing. It should be noted that the steady flow of blood is interupted at curves of the artery wall, e.g. the aortic arch and near branches. At these locations shear stress may fall considerably: there may be turbulent blood flow and even recirculation of blood over certain regions of endothelium. Frequently these locations are the sites where atherosclerotic lesions develop i.e. lesion prone sites.

It is not yet known which protein or proteins are responsible for mechanotransduction ie responsible for responding to changes in a mechanical signal such as shear stress with a biochemical response or responses. Possible **shear stress receptors** include integrins, ion channels, G-protein linked receptors and mitogen activated receptors.

The importance of shear stress in regulating endothelial homeostasis is reflected by the fact that certain genes contain the **shear stress response element** and are thus regulated by changes in shear stress. These include the genes encoding for the following proteins: endothelial nitric oxide synthase, intracellular adhesion molecule ICAM-1 and monocyte chemotactic protein. These proteins have a significant role in the development of atherosclerosis. Another protein affected by shear stress is thrombomodulin, an integral plasma membrane glycoprotein which binds thrombin and thus influences the development of thrombi. The expression of mRNA for thrombomodulin is decreased by increasing shear stress in bovine arterial endothelial cells. Shear stress also has further anticoagulant activity through it's effects upon tissue plasminogen activator and tissue plasminogen activator inhibitor and it's effects upon prostacyclin and nitric oxide release.

6.5 Biochemistry of the intima in atherosclerosis

Nitric oxide

There is a fine balance between the protective activity of nitric oxide and its potential injurious activity.

In atherosclerosis nitric oxide mediated vessel relaxation is impaired. This does not seem to be the result of reduced synthesis of nitric oxide but of a reduction in the effective concentration of nitric oxide by increased reaction with superoxide and lipid peroxyl radicals, both of which are increased in atherosclerotic vessels. This is supported experimentally: eg. intravenous injection of superoxide dismutase, in liposomes to effect entry into the endothelium, can restore the nitric oxide mediated relaxation response to acetylcholine in aorta rings from hypercholesterolemic rabbits.

Nitric oxide reacts with superoxide to produce **peroxynitrite**. This molecule has a short half life, about 1 sec., as it is rapidly protonated at physiological pH to yield the highly reactive peroxynitrous acid which can decompose yielding the nitrate anion, NO_3^- which is physiologically unremarkable. However, peroxynitrite itself is very reactive and is capable of oxidising amino acids, lipids and nucleic acids and of stimulating membrane lipid peroxidation. Peroxynitrite may be the harmful derivative of nitric oxide which has a role in the pathogenesis of atherosclerosis, either through the oxidation of LDL and the ensuing consequences of foam cell formation and/or through the formation of nitrotyrosine. The intermediates of peroxynitrite decomposition are hydroxyl free radical and nitrogen dioxide.

$$O2^- + NO^\bullet \rightarrow ONOO^- + H^+ \rightarrow ONOOH \rightarrow HO^\bullet + NO_2^\bullet \rightarrow NO_3^- + H^+$$

The hydroxyl radical can oxidise lipids (see chapter 9) and the nitrogen dioxide can nitrosylate amino acid such as tyrosine. Thus evidence for the formation of peroxynitrite is obtained by detecting the occurrence of **nitrotyrosine**. Antibodies have been raised to nitrated protein which specifically recognise the nitrotyrosine residue and using these antibodies this "footprint" of peroxynitrite has been observed in the endothelium and lesions of atherosclerotic arteries. Very little nitrated LDL is found in normal aorta but LDL isolated from atherosclerotic aorta does contain nitrotyrosine suggesting that peroxynitrite may be involved in LDL oxidation *in vivo*. However, nitrotyrosine may also be the result of an alternative mechanism involving HOCl. The latter can be produced by macrophages by ***myeloperoxidase***. Evidence of the activity of this enzyme in atherosclerotic lesions is the presence of 3-chlorotyrosine in LDL isolated from these lesions.

It is not known if the presence of nitrotyrosine in proteins is merely the reflection of peroxynitrite presence or whether it has a role in the pathological process. However, the latter seems likely as nitration of functionally important tyrosine residues could profoundly affect homeostasis in one or more of the following ways:

a) inhibition of tyrosine phosphorylation and thus interference with signal transduction,
b) alteration of enzyme and/or cytoskeletal protein conformation and function,
c) may act as a label to induce proteolysis,
d) may initiate the autoimmune process,
e) could act on zinc thiolate centres in transcription factors and modify gene expression.

As mentioned above (6.4) inhibition of the basal nitric oxide production, in cultured endothelial cells, increased the expression of mRNA for monocyte chemotactic protein and increased the secretion of the protein. If this applies *in vivo* the regions of low shear stress where nitric oxide production is low will have a higher rate of secretion of monocyte chemotactic protein than the adjacent endothelium. One of the characteristics of atherosclerosis-prone regions of the artery wall is their exposure to low shear stress. Low nitric oxide production would also favour a higher rate of macrophage colony stimulating factor: nitric oxide inhibits the expression of this growth factor in human endothelial cells in culture. This growth factor stimulates macrophage proliferation and also induces proinflammatory cytokines and cell adhesion molecules. Macrophage colony stimulating factor expression has been observed in human atherosclerotic vessels and the factor was observed to stimulate the expression of the scavenger receptor in human monocytes. Thus low nitric oxide production or a low effective concentration of nitric oxide would facilitate monocyte binding to the endothelium, promote monocyte migration, increase macrophage proliferation and, in the presence of a high concentration of LDL, promote foam cell and fatty streak formation in the intima.

Reduction in effective nitric oxide concentration, in atherosclerosis, reduces its protective effect as an antioxidant thus exacerbating lipoprotein oxidation, reduces the supressive effect on monocyte chemotactic protein synthesis thus favouring more monocyte recruitment to the atherosclerotic lesion, reduces the supressive effect on macrophage colony stimulating factor permitting proliferation of macrophages, and removes or reduces the inhibition of platelet adherence and aggregation, so favouring thrombosis. A further way in which the reduction in effective nitric oxide concentration can increase the atherosclerotic process is that smooth muscle cell proliferation and migration will no longer be inhibited. Direct evidence for a role of nitric oxide in the suppression of smooth muscle proliferation and migration was obtained by transfecting an endothelial nitric oxide synthase gene, *in vivo*, to rat carotid arteries which were denuded of endothelium by balloon injury. This experimental procedure increased nitric oxide production and prevented the neointimal hyperplasia, i.e. new growth of intima, which normally follows this injury.

Endothelin

Endothelin is increased in plasma in symtomatic atherosclerosis. Tumours of the vascular endothelium are associated with high blood pressure. Conversely, anti-endothelin antibody or endothelin receptor antagonists lower blood pressure in animals. The function of endothelin-1 in hypertension and the development of atherosclerosis, in man, has not been established. However it could have a role in progression of atheroma as it does have growth promoting activity.

Growth factors and cytokines

The synthesis of the cytokine, monocyte chemotatic protein and of the growth factor, macrophage colony stimulating factor, in the early stages of atherogenesis has already been described. As the atherosclerotic lesion develops from a fatty streak to an atheroma a number of changes occur in the intima. More monocytes are recruited, more foam cells develop, macrophages and smooth muscle cells proliferate and more extracellular matrix is laid down. In addition T-lymphocytes infiltrate the lesion. The progression of the lesion has features in common with chronic inflammation.

Many of the events in the progression of atherosclerosis are probably the consequence of interaction between cells of the lesion via growth factors, some of which are produced in response to oxidised LDL. The sequence of events is difficult to ascertain especially as some of the actions of growth factors have been observed in culture and their role *in vivo* is less clear. Several of the growth factors are expressed in atherosclerotic lesions but are not seen in the normal artery wall.

Macrophages synthesise various growth factors, notably platelet derived growth factor, (PDGF), interleukin-1α (IL-1 α) and tumour necrosis factor α (TNF α). The latter two growth factors can stimulate endothelial proliferation and like PDGF they also stimulate smooth muscle cell proliferation.

Smooth muscle cells of the synthetic phenotype are capable of expressing genes for a number of growth factors and growth factor receptors and responding to exogenous growth factors. These cells also are responsible for the synthesis of new extracellular matrix proteins and proteoglycans during the progression of atherosclerosis.

T cells are observed in most atherosclerotic lesions in humans. These cells appear to be activated and are thus involved in an immune response. Although the precise antigen responsible for the activation of the T cells within the arterial lesion is uncertain, it may be the oxidised lipoprotein.

6.6 Thrombosis and thrombolysis

Thrombosis

When an atherosclerotic lesion ruptures the sub-endothelial layer is exposed to the blood and a series of normal protective biochemical reactions occur in attempt to close the rupture: coagulation occurs, platelets aggregate and a **thrombus** forms. This is a solid mass containing platelets enmeshed in the polymeric insoluble protein, fibrin. The latter is formed by the action of the enzyme thrombin on the soluble precursor, fibrinogen. This is the last step of the coagulation cascade (see figure6.3). Some thrombi are not life threatening and become incorporated into the atherosclerotic plaque as the initial rupture heals. However if the thrombus occludes (blocks) the artery then thrombosis results. **Thrombosis** is the name given to the clinical condition when formation of a thrombus results in the closure of a vessel leading to ischaemia, i.e. reduced oxygen supply to the surrounding tissues. Thus coronary thrombosis is the condition underlying heart attack (myocardial infarct).

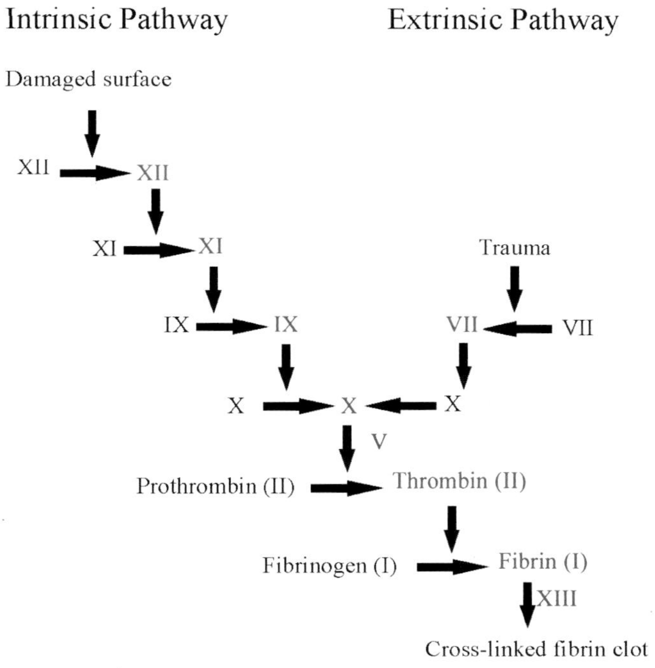

Intrinsic Pathway
Extrinsic Pathway
Damaged surface
XII → XII
XI → XI
IX → IX
Trauma
VII ← VII
X → X ← X
V
Prothrombin (II) → Thrombin (II)
Fibrinogen (I) → Fibrin (I)
XIII
Cross-linked fibrin clot

Figure 6.3
Blood clotting cascade illustrating the role of thrombin

Molecules in red are activated forms of clotting factors: several of these are serine proteases. Each activated clotting factor stimulates the activation of another factor in the cascade.

Thrombosis rarely occurs in the presence of a healthy and undamaged endothelium. The basal secretions of the healthy endothelial cells are mainly anti-coagulant. Formation of thrombin affects the endothelium and some pro-coagulationary secretions may be promoted (see table 6. 2). However some of the interactions of thrombin with the endothelium limit the activity of this enzyme (see table 6.2).

Thrombolysis

The reactions of thrombolysis, i.e. dispersal of thrombi, prevent undesirable formation of thrombi in flowing blood and limit the growth of a thrombus when formed at the site of an injury. Natural thrombolysis is seen in patients after heart attacks. Immediately after myocardial infarct most patients show evidence of blockage of a coronary artery, when the coronary arteriograms were examined, whereas several hours later such thrombi often disperse.

Treatment of patients with myocardial infarct with **thrombolytic agents** reduces the subsequent mortality of these patients and has become routine treatment in many coronary care units contributing to the reduced incidence of death from coronary heart disease that has been seen in the past two decades.

Several major epidemiological trials established the efficacy of three thrombolytic agents: *streptokinase*, an enzyme from *Haemolytic streptoccoci*, recombinant tissue plasminogen activator and anisoylated plasminogen-streptokinase activator complex. Administration of aspirin, which has anti-platelet activity, enhances the effect of these thrombolytic agents.

6.7 Conclusion

In simple terms atherosclerosis, which is a disease of the intima of the artery wall, may be caused by a disturbance of homeostasis in the artery wall ie. by some disruption of the normal interactions within and between cells and the intracellular matrix of the intima. The risk factors, hypertension and hypercholesteroemia may separately produce disruption, and together more profoundly disturb homeostasis, and hence can be regarded as causes of the disease. Prolonging the period of exposure of the artery wall to either or both conditions will enhance progression of the disease by continued disturbance of homeostasis.

The initial formation of foam cells may represent a normal response to a disturbance of homeostasis: too much lipoprotein, oxidation of this and the need to remove the oxidised lipid from the intima by recruited monocytes which have differentiated into macrophages. However the persistance of conditions which have favoured foam cell formation may

Table 6.2 Effects of thrombin on endothelial cells (adapted from Pearson, 1994)

Biochemical effect	*Biochemical response*	*Comment*
Reactions which promote thrombosis		
Promotes synthesis and secretion of **tissue factor**	Initiates blood coagulation	Release of this factor signals the initiation of coagulation cascade. Synthesis of this factor is normally repressed
Increased synthesis and secretion of **von Willibrand factor**	Cofactor required for efficient platelet adhesion to extracellular matrix	Released in response to local tissue injury to facilitate formation of haemostatic plug ie a thrombus.
Increases **P selectin** expression	This protein enhances neutrophil adhesion to endothelial cells	Neutrophils may enter intima in atherosclerosis and inflammation
Reactions which promote thrombolysis		
Increases synthesis and secretion of **tissue plasminogen activator** (tPA) and **plasminogen activator inhibitor** (PAi-I)	PAi-I is normally in excess, forms a complex with tPA and the complex is cleared from the blood. tPA stimulates the conversion of plasminogen to plasmin, the enzyme which hydrolyses fibrin	tPA promotes thrombolysis
Increased synthesis and secretion of **prostaglandin**	Inhibits platelet aggregation, promotes vasodilation	Limits growth of intravascular thrombus
Increased synthesis and secretion of **nitric oxide**	Inhibits platelet aggregation, promotes vasodilation.	Limits growth of intravascular thrombus May act synergistically with prostaglandin *in vivo*.
Reaction with **antithrombin** on endothelial membrane	The antithrombin-thrombin complex dissociates and is cleared from the blood by the liver	Reduction in active thrombin
Reaction with **thrombomodulin**	Properties of thrombin change when bound to endothelial surface -thrombomodulin	Reduced action on fibrinogen. Activation of protein C, which inactivates factors V and VIII and PAi-I

cause further development, with more foam cell formation, involvement of smooth muscle cells in lipid accumulation and fatty streaks formation. Progression to more advanced lesions requires further participation of smooth muscle cells, proliferation of these and increased synthesis of extra cellular matrix components by these cells.

HDL may prevent the development and the progression of atherosclerosis by removing cholesterol from the intima or by preventing the oxidation of LDL.

Clinical symptoms of atherosclerotic disease begin when atherosclerotic lesions reduce blood flow and impair oxygen supply to tissue. Dangerous, life threatening conditions arise when atherosclerotic lesions rupture or fissure and thrombosis occurs. To avoid this measures need to be taken to stabilise lesions to prevent their damage and to promote regression where this is possible. The regression of atherosclerosis is discussed in chapter 11.

Key references

General

Schwartz, C.J., Valente, A.J. and Sprague, E.A. (1993) A modern view of atherogenesis. American Journal of Cardiology 71, 9B-14B

Williams, K.J. and Tabas, I. (1995) The response to retention hypothesis of early atherogenesis. Arteriosclerosis Thrombosis and Vascular Biology 15, 551-561

Camejo, G. *et al.* (1998) Association of apoB lipoproteins with arterial proteoglycans: pathological significance and molecular basis. Atherosclerosis 139, 205-222

Transendothelial transport of LDL

Schwenke, D.C. and Carew, T.E. (1989) Initiation of atherosclerotic lesions in cholesterol-fed rabbits. Arteriosclerosis 9,895-907

Nielson, L.B. (1996) Transfer of low density lipoproteins into the arterial wall and risk of atherosclerosis. Atherosclerosis 123, 1-15

Foam cell formation: LDL modification, LDL oxidation and the scavenger receptor

Holvoet, P. and Collen, D. (1994) Oxidised lipoproteins in atherosclerosis and thrombosis. FASEB Journal. 8, 1279-1284

Berliner, J.A. *et al.* (1995) Atherosclerosis: basic mechanisms. oxidation, inflammation and genetics. Circulation 91, 2488-2496

Steinberg, D. (1997) Low density lipoprotein oxidation and its pathological significance. Journal of Biological Chemistry 272, 20963-20966

HDL and atheroma

Navab, M. *et al.* (1996) The yin and yang of oxidation in the development of the fatty streak. Arteriosclerosis Thrombosis and Vascular Biology 16, 831-842

Nitric oxide

Fleming, I. and Busse, R. (1995) Control and consequences of endothelial nitric oxide formation. Advances in Pharmacology 34, 187-206

Luoma, J. *et al.* (1998) Expression of extracellular SOD and iNOS in macrophages and smooth muscle cells in human and rabbit atherosclerotic lesions: colocalisation with epitopes characteristic of oxidised LDL and peroxynitrite modified proteins. Arteriosclerosis Thrombosis and Vascular Biology 18, 157-167

Endothelin

Masaki, T. (1995) Possible role of endothelin in endothelial regulation of vascular tone. Annual Reviews of Pharmacology and Toxicology 35, 235-255

Shear stress

Davies, P.F. (1995) Flow mediated endothelial mechanotransduction. Physiological Reviews 75, 519-560

Traub, O. and Berk, B.C. (1998) Laminar shear stress. Mechanisms by which endothelial cells transduce atheroprotective force. Arterio-sclerosclerosis Thrombosis and Vascular Biology 18, 677-685

Growth factors and cytokines

Ross, R. (1993) The pathogenesis of atherosclerosis: a perspective for the 1990s. Nature 362, 801-809

Thrombosis and thrombolysis

Pearson, J.D. (1994) Vessel wall interactions regulating thrombosis. British Medical Bulletin 50, 776-788

7 Dietary Cholesterol and Fat

7.1 Introduction

Human intakes of dietary fat vary enormously. Agricultural communities of the third world may be consuming as little as 10% of their total energy intake as fat, while in Western industrialised countries this may be as high as 50%. Generally, a high fat intake is associated with large amounts of animal tissue in the diets. Such tissues, particularly red meats from ruminant animals, tend to be rich in saturated fatty acids. As will be discussed below, a vast amount of evidence exists to suggest that a high intake of saturated fat is associated with elevated plasma cholesterol concentrations, and hence increased risk of coronary heart disease (CHD). However, it is important not to look at saturated fat intake in isolation. The high saturated fat intake, but low incidence of CHD in hunter-gather populations such as the Masai tribe of Kenya is often quoted as evidence against a role of saturated fat. Clearly, as with all aspect of cardiovascular disease, other dietary, environmental and genetic factors must be taken into account when considering the potential influence of dietary factors on risk of developing CHD.

A popular misconception is that all animal fats are bad and all vegetable oils are good. While there is a large range of vegetable oils which are rich in monounsaturated or polyunsaturated fatty acids there are others such as coconut oil and palm oil which are made up almost entirely of saturated fatty acids. Dietary intake of the saturated plant oils is surprisingly high due their use in processed foods. Furthermore, the process of hydrogenation to form solid fats from vegetable oils not only increases their saturated fatty acid content but also produces, potentially harmful *trans* fatty acids.

One continuing area of confusion to the general public is the effect of dietary cholesterol on CHD risk. It appears obviously straight- forward that eating cholesterol increases plasma cholesterol. As such, many people believe that it is the cholesterol content of meat rather than the fat content that is the problem. However, as we shall see below, under normal conditions dietary cholesterol intake probably has only a modest effect on plasma cholesterol levels. The source of cholesterol in the diet is also often a point of confusion, with many people believing that meat and diary produce are the foods which contribute most. In fact, for most of us there is only one significant source of cholesterol in the diet, namely hen's eggs. A single hen's egg can contain 200-300mg of cholesterol. With most peoples dietary intakes rarely exceeding 500mg/day, with the wide use of eggs, not only as a primary food but also used in the production of a vast array of processed foods, it is clear that the egg is by far the principle source of dietary cholesterol.

7.2 Fatty acids in the diet

Structure of fatty acids

As already stated in chapter 4, fatty acids are hydrocarbon chains with terminal methyl and carboxyl groups. There are a large number of fatty acids occurring in nature which differ in chain length, number of double bonds, position of double bonds and type of double bonds. However, there are probably less than twenty that are quantitatively important in the human diet, with two (palmitic acid and oleic acid) often accounting for more than 65% of total fatty acid intake. Table 7.1 describes the more commonly occurring fatty acids, dividing them into the classes saturated (SFA), monounsaturated (MUFA) and polyunsaturated (PUFA) fatty acids depending on the presence and number of double bonds.

Table 7.1
Common dietary fatty acids and their sources

Fatty acid	*Formula*	*Typical intake (g/day)*	*Some common sources*
Saturated			
Medium chain	C6:0-C10:0	2	Coconut oil, Butter fat
Lauric	C12:0	2	Coconut oil, palm kernel oil
Myristic	C14:0	8	Coconut oil, palm kernel oil, dairy products
Palmitic	C16:0	30	Dairy products, meat, palm oil
Stearic	C18:0	15	Cocoa butter, meat
Monounsaturated			
Oleic	C18:1cis	32	Meat, olive & rapeseed oil
Elaidic	C18:1trans	6	Hydrogenated fats
Polyunsaturated			
Linoleic	C18:2 (n-6)	12	Sunflower, corn & safflower oils
Gamma -linolenic	C18:3 (n-6)	0.1	Evening primrose oil
Alpha -linolenic	C18:3 (n-3)	2	Linseed oil, soybean oil, vegetables
Eicosapentanoic	C20:5 (n-3)	0.3	Fish, marine mammals
Docosahexaenoic	C20:5 (n-3)	0.1	Fish, marine mammals

Occurrence of dietary fatty acids

In excess of 95% of total dietary intake of fatty acids is in the form of triacylglycerol (TAG) (see chapter 4). Most natural food sources contain a wide variety of saturated and unsaturated fatty acids and thus a large number of TAG molecules of different fatty acid composition. Lard, for example, would be considered by many people as being a saturated fat. However, over 40% of the fatty acid content is oleic acid and 10% is linoleic acid. On the other hand, olive oil, generally regarded as a monounsaturated oil, actually contains 12% palmitic acid.

Essential fatty acids

Dietary fatty acids fulfil three major roles; an energy source, structural components of membranes and precursors to other molecules. The first of these functions cannot be described as essential. Dietary fat represents a convenient energy-rich food source, the consumption of which reduces the time we spend eating and the volume of food required. However, the role of fatty acids as energy providers can be adequately fulfilled by carbohydrate. Furthermore, energy consumed as carbohydrate in excess of immediate requirements can be converted into fatty acids for storage within adipose tissue. The major proportions of fatty acids that are found in membranes are also not essential. Palmitic acid, stearic acid and oleic acid can all be made *de novo* through the actions of *fatty acid synthase*, *fatty acid elongase* and *stearoyl CoA desaturase* respectively. However, linoleic acid (C18:2 n-6) and alpha -linolenic acid (C18:3 n-3) cannot be made by animals and are thus essential components of the diet. This appears to be a result of their requirements in the membranes and as precursors of the eicosanoids. Essential Fatty Acid (EFA) deficiency results in a variety of symptoms which include increased permeability of membranes to water and small molecules which directly relates to changes in the fatty acid composition of the membranes. In addition the inability to synthesise eicosanoids such as thromboxanes, prostaglandins, prostacyclins and leukotrienes in EFA deficiency leads to a wide range of physiological disturbances.

7.3 Effects of dietary cholesterol and fat on plasma cholesterol

The Keys and Hegsted equations

It is over 30 years since Keys *et al* (1965) and, working independently, Hegsted *et al* (1965) derived predictive equations to quantify the effects of dietary cholesterol and fat on plasma cholesterol concentrations. These equations (table 7.2) were derived from regression analysis from a large number of human feeding trials in which the amount of cholesterol, saturated and polyunsaturated fatty acids were manipulated.

While there are minor quantitative differences between the two equations, the overall conclusions were similar:

Table 7.2 Equations for predicting the effect of dietary cholesterol and/or fatty acids on plasma and lipoprotein cholesterol concentrations

Authors	*Year*	*Equations*
Keys *et al*	1965	$\Delta Ch = (0.0708\Delta S - 0.0339\Delta P) + \sqrt{\Delta C}$ *ΔCh = change in plasma cholesterol (mmol/l)* *ΔS & ΔP = change in % calories from saturated & polyunsaturated fatty acids respectively* *ΔC = change in dietary cholesterol (mg/1000 kcal)*
Hegsted *et al*	1965	$\Delta Ch = (0.0558\Delta S - 0.0426\Delta P) + (0.0651\Delta C) - 0.53$ *As above except; ΔC = change in dietary cholesterol (mg/day)*
Mensink & Katan	1992	ΔCh = 0.039(carb® sat) - 0.003(carb® mono) - 0.015(carb® poly) ΔLDL = 0.033(carb® sat) - 0.006(carb® mono) - 0.014(carb® poly) ΔHDL = 0.012(carb® sat) + 0.009(carb® mono) + 0.007(carb® poly) *Where ΔLDL and ΔHDL represent the change in total plasma cholesterol, LDL cholesterol or HDL cholesterol (mmol/l) respectively* *carb® sat, carb® mono and carb® poly represent the change in % energy as carbohydratereplaced by saturated, monounsaturated or polyunsaturated fatty acids respectively*
Hegsted *et al*	1993	$\Delta Ch = 0.0543\Delta S - 0.0301\Delta P + 0.00725\Delta C$ $\Delta LDL = 0.0449\Delta S - 0.0198\Delta P + 0.00475\Delta C$ $\Delta HDL = 0.0110\Delta S + 0.0056\Delta P + 0.0026\Delta M + 0.0047\Delta C$ *ΔS, ΔP& ΔM = change in % calories from saturated, polyunsaturated andmonounsaturated fatty acids respectively. ΔC = change in dietary cholesterol (J/kg)*
Yu *et al*	1993	ΔCh = 0.0522Δ12:0 - 16:0 - 0.0008Δ18:0 - 0.0124ΔM - 0.0248ΔP ΔLDL = 0.0378Δ12:0-16:0 - 0.0018Δ18:0 - 0.0178ΔM - 0.0248ΔP ΔHDL = 0.0160Δ12:0-16:0 - 0.0016Δ18:0 + 0.0101ΔM + 0.0062ΔP *Where Δ12:0-16:0 represents change in % energy for lauric, myristic & palmitic acid and Δ18:0 change in % energy from stearic acid*

See Key References for further details

1) Dietary cholesterol has a relatively modest plasma cholesterol raising effect
2) Dietary saturated fatty acids have a potent cholesterol-raising effect
3) Dietary polyunsaturated fatty acids (PUFA) have a plasma cholesterol-reducing effect.
4) The cholesterol-raising effect of saturated fatty acids is more potent than the cholesterol-lowering effects of polyunsaturated fatty acids.

Recent meta-analyses

Despite a vast number of human feeding studies since the derivation of these equations these major conclusions have withstood the test of time remarkably well. However, as our knowledge of the role of lipoproteins in the development of premature cardiovascular disease has increased it has become apparent that there is a need to distinguish effect of diet on low-density lipoprotein (LDL) cholesterol from those on high-density lipoprotein (HDL) cholesterol. Furthermore, increasing interest has focused on the effects of specific fatty acids rather than broad classes based on degree of saturation. As a result, in recent years a number of attempts have been made to develop predictive equations that take into account these factors. One technique that has been used is that of meta-analysis. This statistical tool is used to pool results from a number of different trials in order to increase the statistical power of the data. Having set specific criteria of the inclusion, or exclusion of data from the analysis a careful survey of published literature is performed to gather together the relevant studies.

Mensink and Katan (1992) analysed 27 well-controlled trials on dietary fatty acids and plasma lipoproteins. The resulting equations are shown in table 7.2. In terms of effects on total plasma cholesterol the results tended to confirm the findings of Keys and Hegsted. One difference, however, was that monounsaturated fatty acids (MUFA), of which oleic acid is quantitatively the most important, were found to have a modest cholesterol lowering effect. This is in contrast to the earlier studies that regarded MUFA as equivalent to carbohydrate and hence omitted them from regression equations. Saturated fatty acids (SFA) increase both LDL and HDL cholesterol but the effect on the former is substantially greater. PUFA decrease LDL to a greater extent, but increase HDL to a slightly lesser extent, than do MUFA. This data contradicts certain reports that suggest PUFA may actually reduce HDL cholesterol. It has been suggested that such an effect only occur at very high PUFA concentrations that would not normally occur in the human diet. Surprisingly, these results indicated that replacing saturated fatty acids with unsaturated fatty acids was actually more beneficial than replacing them with carbohydrate. This casts some doubt on any advice to simply reduce total fat intake without altering the nature of the fat eaten.

A similar meta-analysis was performed in 1993 by Hegsted *et al* (table 7.2). Data included 420 dietary observations from 141 different groups of subjects. In addition to looking at the effect of dietary fatty acids they also re-evaluated the effect of dietary cholesterol itself. In contrast to the findings of Mensink and Katan dietary MUFA were judged to have no significant influence on either total or LDL cholesterol concentrations and were therefore omitted from the equations. A modest, but significant contribution of dietary cholesterol to the increase in total cholesterol was confirmed and this was found to be true for LDL cholesterol as well. Dietary cholesterol, SFA, MUFA and PUFA all tended to increase plasma HDL cholesterol but the regression coefficients were only statistically significant for SFA and MUFA. Overall the equation derived was a poor fit for the data and the authors concluded that changes in HDL cholesterol could not be satisfactorily predicted from the data available. Like Mensink and Katan they showed that there was little evidence of a beneficial effect of changing total fat intake without changing fatty acid composition.

The conflicting views of Mensink and Katan (1992) and Hegsted *et al* (1993) on the effects of MUFA on total and lipoprotein cholesterol were addressed in another recent meta-analysis (Gardner & Kraemer, 1995). This analysis looked specifically at studies where MUFA and PUFA were directly exchanged without significant changes in total and saturated fat or dietary cholesterol. Fourteen such studies, performed between 1983-1994 were identified. The overall conclusion of this analysis was that there was no significant difference between the effects of MUFA and PUFA on total, LDL or HDL cholesterol but that PUFA produced a modest reduction in plasma triacylglycerol. It was suggested that the disagreement between this study and those of Keys *et al* (1965) and Hegsted *et al* (1965) as regards the relative effects of MUFA and PUFA may relate to the type of feeding study considered. While these previous studies looked at dietary manipulation where significant changes in total and saturated fat and dietary cholesterol occurred, Gardner & Kramer limited themselves to those in which all of these variables were kept constant and only MUFA and PUFA were inter-changed.

Perhaps the most ambitious attempt to quantify the effects of dietary fatty acids on plasma lipoprotein concentrations is the analysis reported by Yu *et al* (1995). They used 18 published studies to perform meta-analysis on the effects of individual fatty acids on plasma total, LDL and HDL cholesterol in men and women. The overall equations for both sexes combined are shown in table 7.2.

One of the major differences between the analysis by Yu *et al* (1995) and previous analyses is that it includes stearic acid (C18.0) which in the past has tended to be included with other saturates or regarded as neutral. The latter was confirmed in the present study where none of the correlation coefficients for stearic acid were significantly different from zero. Generally, the predictive changes for total and LDL cholesterol were similar for men and women; however interesting sex differences were seen in the response of HDL cholesterol. The response to both stearic acid and PUFA were different between the sexes with both significantly reducing HDL cholesterol in women compared to men.

As with the original Keys and Hegsted equations quantitative differences exist in the more recent analyses described above. Furthermore, disagreement still prevails over the effects of MUFA. However, again some common conclusions can be drawn.

1) Saturated fats increase LDL and HDL cholesterol but have their greatest effect on LDL
2) MUFA and PUFA probably both decrease LDL cholesterol
3) Except at exceptionally high intakes, PUFA does not decrease HDL and MUFA may actually increase it
4) Stearic acid has an essentially neutral effect on total plasma cholesterol
5) There is little evidence to suggest that moderate changes in total fat intake without a change in fatty acid composition has any beneficial effects on total cholesterol and might actually produce a more detrimental lipoprotein profile.

Comparative effects of different saturated fatty acids

The equations discussed above appear to show that not all saturated fatty acids are equally potent at raising plasma cholesterol. Hegsted originally reported myristic acid as being four times more hypercholesterolaemic as palmitic acid. The more recent meta-analyses also appear to support this finding. By contrast, lauric and palmitic acid appear to be equally potent at raising cholesterol.

Not all human feeding trials support these results from meta-analysis. In general most studies which have directly compared the effects of diets specifically enriched in either myristic or palmitic acids tend to show that the cholesterol-raising effects of these fatty acids are much more similar than suggested by the meta-analyses described above. This appears to be the case whether the fats used are derived from natural sources or whether they are artificially produced. The reason for this discrepancy remains to be established.

The lack of effect of stearic acid on plasma cholesterol has been confirmed in a number of human feeding trials. What remains to be established is why this should be the case. Ideas that have been suggested include the poor absorption of stearic acid from the gut, it's desaturation to oleic acid in the intestine, adipose tissue or liver or specific differences in the metabolism of stearic acid compared to the other long-chain saturated fatty acids. It is likely that a combination of these factors contribute to it'' "neutrality".

Trans fatty acids

Fatty acids containing double bonds in the *trans*, as opposed to the *cis* configuration occur relatively rarely in nature. The action of bacteria in the rumen creates some such fatty acids that then can accumulate in the tissues and milk of ruminant animals. However, the major source of *trans* fatty acids is processed oils and fats, such as margarine. Such foods can contain appreciable amounts of *trans* C18:1 (elaidic acid) and lesser amounts of a range of polyunsaturated fatty acids containing various combinations of *cis* and *trans* double bonds. Concerns over the potential effect of such fatty acids have been voiced over a number of years though earlier data was judged to be inconclusive. However, data emerging from the recent American Nurses Study has renewed such concern. This study amassed dietary histories from 85,095 subjects and showed a stronger link between CHD and *trans* fatty acid consumption, than with saturated fatty acid intake.

Unfortunately insufficient data is available to perform meta-analysis on *trans* fatty acid intake of a similar manner to that performed on other types of fatty acid. However, the results of recent well controlled human feeding studies do support the idea that the increased risk of CHD described above may be the result of adverse changes in plasma lipoprotein cholesterol concentrations. Most of the data available suggests that trans fatty acids may specifically increase LDL cholesterol, decrease HDL cholesterol and also increased Lp(a) concentrations. This has led to calls for drastic cuts in the amount of *trans* fatty acid being consumed. What remains to be firmly established is the relative effect of elaidic acid and saturated fatty acids. It would seem imprudent, at the present time, to recommend changes in dietary habits which exchange hydrogenated fats for those rich in lauric, myristic or palmitic acid. The effects of PUFAs containing *trans* double bonds, at the relatively low concentrations at which they occur, also remain to be established.

n-3 polyunsaturated fatty acids

The n-3, or omega 3, polyunsaturated fatty acids represent a class of polyunsaturates in which the first double bond occurs after the third, rather than the more common sixth (n-6), carbon from the methyl end of the fatty acid. While these fatty acids are relatively rare in the tissues of animals they are more common in certain plant oils (e.g. linseed oil) and within the tissues of certain organisms of marine origin.

Much interest has focused around the potentially beneficial effect of fish oils, rich in eicosapentaenoic acid (EPA, C20:5) and docosahexaenoic acid (DHA, C22:6). This relates to findings that coastal populations, such as Greenland Eskimos have an incidence of CHD as low as 8% of that of comparable inland populations. Such communities habitually consume a diet containing 7g/day of marine n-3 fatty acids compared to 0.06g/day in most Western diets. Compared to age and sex matched Danes, these Eskimos were found to have lower total, very low density lipoprotein (VLDL) and LDL cholesterol and higher HDL cholesterol concentrations. This has led to numerous studies of the effects of diets enriched in oily fish or supplemented with fish oils. In 1989 Harris reviewed the more well controlled studies performed up to that date. The overall effect on total and LDL in normolipaemic subjects was judged to be negligible. A slight rise, or 3%, in HDL cholesterol was calculated. However plasma triacylglycerol concentrations were much more dramatically affected with a 25% decrease. The overall conclusion of this analysis was that, while fish oils have a marked triacylglycerol-lowering effect, there was little to suggest significant beneficial changes in total LDL or HDL cholesterol concentrations. Thus, it is likely that any protective effects of fish-oil consumption or cardiovascular risk relate to other risk factors such as platelet function, blood pressure, blood flow, inflammatory processes and the atherogenic process itself.

7.4 Mechanisms whereby dietary fatty acids may influence plasma cholesterol concentrations

Fatty acid incorporation into VLDL

Fatty acids of both endogenous and exogenous origin can be incorporated into triacylglycerol and phospholipid destined for incorporation into VLDL. Different fatty acids appear to be specifically channelled into the synthesis of these lipids. The incorporation of triacylglycerol and cholesterol into VLDL appears to be co-ordinately regulated and thus the metabolic fate of different fatty acids in the liver may influence their effect on VLDL secretion and ultimately LDL production.

Regulation of hepatic sterol metabolism

Cholesterol, or one of its metabolites, can alter hepatic gene expression *via* the sterol regulatory element (see chapter 4). It has been proposed that it is by altering the distribution of cholesterol between various pools within the liver that fatty acids exert many of their effects on cholesterol metabolism. Detailed studies by Spady, Dietschy and co-workers indicate that saturated fatty acids of 12, 14 and 16 carbon atoms decrease LDL receptor activity and increase LDL production rate with a consequent increase in plasma LDL levels. These workers suggest that it is by regulating the size of this cholesterol ester pool, and thereby the pool of sterol that regulates LDL receptor activity, that dietary fatty acids exert their effect. Thus, long chain SFA may decrease the storage of hepatic cholesterol ester, increase the size of the regulatory pool and down-regulate LDL receptors. By contrast oleic acid appears to actively increase the cholesterol ester pool thereby decreasing the amount of "regulatory cholesterol" and hence up regulates LDL receptor expression. Finally other fatty acids such as shorter chain SFA (C4-10), elaidic and linoleic acid appear to be essentially neutral in this process.

Dietary fats and gene expression

Another possibility is that dietary fatty acids may act by directly influencing the expression of genes associated with lipoprotein metabolism. Evidence is accumulating that fatty acids may act as important modulators of the expression of transcription factors such as the peroxisomal proliferator activated receptor and the hepatic nuclear factors, which may then interact with the promoters of genes coding for proteins including various apolipoproteins, enzymes and lipoprotein receptors.

7.5 Conclusions

Early work firmly established a link between the quantity and quality of dietary fat and plasma cholesterol concentrations. Most dietary recommendations are still based on the outcome of such studies. More recent evidence has suggested specific and unique effects of individual fatty acids on plasma cholesterol and its distribution between the individual lipoprotein classes. Meta-analyses have quantified these effects in such a way that the influence of a particular dietary fat can be predicted from its fatty acid profile. A major challenge for the future is to be able to translate this information into specific, LDL cholesterol - lowering dietary recommendations. It seems unlikely that the interpretation of such data can be left in the hands of the consumer and it may be put to greater use by the oils and fats industry in formulating products.

Major advances have been made in recent years in our understanding of the molecular mechanisms whereby dietary fatty acids are influencing lipoprotein metabolism. It has become quite clear that in addition to their well defined roles in energy metabolism, as constituents of membranes and as precursors to hormones, fatty acids might also directly regulate gene expression. It is appears likely that future research will provide a greater understanding of the mechanisms whereby fatty acids exert many of their regulatory effects on lipoprotein metabolism.

Key references

General

Grundy, S.M. and Denke, M.A. (1990) Dietary influences on serum lipids and lipoproteins. Journal of Lipid Research 31, 1149-1172

Spady, D.K, Woollett, L.A. and Dietschy, J.M. (1993) Regulation of plasma LDL-cholesterol levels by dietary cholesterol and fatty acids. Annual Reviews of Nutrition 13, 355-381

Salter, A.M. and White, D.A. (1996) Effects of dietary fat on cholesterol metabolism: regulation of plasma LDL concentrations. Nutritiition Research Reviews 9, 241-257

n-3 polyunsaturated fatty acids

Harris, W.S. (1989) Fish oils and plasma lipid and lipoprotein metabolism in humans: a critical review. Journal of Lipid Research 30, 785-807

Trans fatty acids

Gurr, M.I. (1996) Dietary fatty acids with trans unsaturation. Nutrition Research Reviews 9, 259-279

Predictive equations

Keys, A. *et al*. (1965) Serum cholesterol response to changes in diet. IV particular saturated fatty acids in the diet. Metabolism 14, 776-787

Hegsted, D.M. *et al*. (1965) Quantitative effects of dietary fat on serum cholesterol in man. American Journal of Clinical Nutrition 17, 281-295

Mensink, R.P. and Katan, M.B. (1992) Effect of dietary fatty acids on lipids and lipoproteins: a meta-analysis of 27 trials. Arteriosclerosis and Thrombosis 12, 911-919

Hegsted, D.M. *et al*. (1993) Dietary fat and serum lipids an evaluation of the experimental data. American Journal of Clinical Nutrition 57, 875-883

S.M. Yu *et al*. (1995) Plasma cholesterol predictive equations demonstrate that stearic acid is neutral and monounsaturated fatty acids are hypocholesterolaemic. American Journal of Clinical Nutrition 61, 1129-1139

Gardner, C.D. and Kraemer, H.C. (1995) Monounsaturated versus polyunsaturated dietary fat and serum lipids. A meta-analysis. Arteriosclerosis, Thrombosis and Vascular Biology 15, 1917-1927

8 Other Macronutrients: Carbohydrates and Proteins

8.1 Introduction

For obvious reasons research into the effects of diet on lipoprotein metabolism and cardiovascular disease has focussed extensively on dietary lipids. The high incidence of coronary heart disease in the Western world is almost certainly closely associated with the very high fat intakes these countries. However, dietary cholesterol and fatty acids are not the only components of the diet that may influence plasma lipoprotein concentrations. In this chapter the influence of other macronutrient constituents of the diet are considered. One important factor to be remembered is that, when dealing with free-living human populations it is almost impossible to consider one aspect of the diet without taking into account other constituents. For example, in populations that are still dependent on "peasant" agriculture much higher levels of dietary carbohydrate and fibre are consumed than in most of the countries of Northern Europe and North America. Most of these countries report much lower incidences of cardiovascular disease. However, such diets are inherently low in dietary fat. So is it the high amounts of carbohydrate, high amounts of fibre or low amounts of fat that are protective? As will be discussed below, evidence exists to suggest that dietary protein of vegetable origin may be "hypocholesterolaemic" compared to that of animal origin. However, animal protein is usually associated with higher intakes of saturated fatty acid and cholesterol. Thus, interpreting results that compare different human populations consuming very different diets and attributing effects to single nutrients can be very difficult. For this reason we are dependent on controlled experiments where the total nutrient content of the diet can be carefully regulated before active effects of individual components can be defined. Furthermore, if we are interested in the mechanism of action of these nutrients, then animal models may represent the only practical system in which to perform such studies.

8.2 Carbohydrates

Evolution of the human diet

In many parts of the world the human diet has changed beyond recognition within the last 10,000 years. Prior to the "Agricultural revolution" human populations existed as "Hunter-Gatherers". Studies of such populations that still exist indicate that they consume a diet low in fat and high in carbohydrate compared to present-day affluent societies. As such 50-70% of energy intake is derived from carbohydrate and 15-20% from fat. This compares with current UK intakes of about 46% carbohydrate and 40% fat. In addition the nature of the carbohydrate intake is very different with the Hunter-Gatherers consuming virtually all of their carbohydrate as starch while almost half of our intake is in the form of simple mono- and di- saccharides. The agricultural revolution led to a more stable food supply but did not significantly change the dietary sources of energy with carbohydrate still supply 60-75%. Even, a mere two hundred years ago in the UK fat intake was only about a sixth of its current level.

These dramatic changes in diet have not of course been accompanied by any biological evolution of the human species. Our digestive and metabolic systems remain much the same as they were in the "hunter-gatherers days". Thus it is hardly surprising that such massive changes in dietary intakes have resulted in dramatic changes in our normal and pathological responses to diet. To what extent can the reduction in carbohydrate intake be associated with our increased susceptibility to cardiovascular disease?

Effect of high carbohydrate diets on lipoprotein metabolism

The major carbohydrates in our diet can be classified as **monosaccharides** and **disaccharides** (commonly referred to as sugars), **polysaccharides** (primarily starch) and non-starch polysaccharides (or fibre). Some of the more common forms of dietary carbohydrate are listed in table 8.1. In the UK, sugars contribute about 18% and starch about 24% of total energy intake. Much of the sugar intake represents extrinsic refined sugar that we have added to our diet. On the other hand dietary fibre contributes little in terms of energy but, as will be discussed below, may still have an important impact on lipoprotein metabolism.

If an individual consuming a typical Western diet rich in total and saturated fat switches to a low fat, high carbohydrate diet then there are rapid effects on plasma lipoprotein concentrations. The main effects appear to be on triacylglycerol concentrations rather than cholesterol, with a significant increase in VLDL triacylglcylcerol. This can, however, also be associated with a decrease in the level of HDL cholesterol. In some individuals these changes may be transient with concentrations returning to normal after a few weeks, while in others they may persist. Animal studies suggest that dietary fructose, or fructose containing - sucrose, induces a greater hypertriglyceridaemic response than glucose or starch. This may relate to difference in the metabolism of fructose and glucose with more of the former being channeled into fatty acid synthesis and esterification. There appears to be little evidence of a similar significant effect in humans.

Table 8.1 Different types of dietary carbohydrates and their sources

Class	*Example*	*Some sources*	*Composition*
Monosaccharide	Glucose	Fruit, honey	
	Fructose	Fruit, Honey	
	Galactose	Component of lactose	
Disaccharide	Sucrose	Cane & beet sugar	α 1,4 -linked glucose & fructose
	Maltose	Sprouted grain	α 1,4 -linked glucose & glucose
	Lactose	Milk	ß 1,4 -linked galactose & glucose
Polysaccharide	Amylopectin (starch)	Cereals	α 1,4 & α 1,6 -linked, branched polymer of glucose
	Amylose (starch)	Cereals	α 1,4 -linked, linear polymer of glucose
	Glycogen (animal starch)	Liver, muscle	α 1,4 & α 1,6 -linked, branched polymer of glucose
Insoluble Fibre	Cellulose	Plant cell walls	ß 1,4 -linked, linear polymers of glucose
Soluble Fibre	Pectin	Fruits	ß 1,4 -linked linear polymer of galactu-ronic acids and/or modified galacturonic acid
	ß-glucan	Cereals	ß 1,3 & ß 1,4 -linked, branched polymers of glucose

Thus, in terms of cardiovascular risk the most important effect of digestible dietary carbohydrates appears to be a potential reduction in HDL cholesterol. In view of the low incidence of cardiovascular disease in countries, which consume high carbohydrate/low fat diets, the relevance of this reduction in HDL remains to be established. It would probably be fair to say that compared to a typical, high-saturated fat, Western diet, a low fat, high carbohydrate-diet would be protective from cardiovascular disease.

8.3 Dietary fibre

Considerable debate has gone on over the years as to what we actually mean by the term dietary fibre. In general, it is used to describe the components of plant cell wall that escape digestion. The largest proportion of such material represents a range of carbohydrates that can be described as "**non-starch polysaccharides**" or **NSP**. While the term dietary fibre is still widely used there have been moves to replace it with the term NSP. For the purposes of the discussion below the terms dietary fibre and NSP are used synonymously and refer to the non-digestible, non-alpha-linked carbohydrate fraction of plant material.

Dietary fibre makes little contribution to energy intake in humans. Animals lack the enzymes that can break the ß-linkages within the carbohydrate chains. Some species, e.g. the ruminants, have overcome this by developing digestive systems that host bacteria that perform the digestion for them. In humans, however, any such symbiosis occurs in the large intestine from where there is little absorption of the products of digestion. Despite this it appears that dietary fibre does have the potential to influence lipoprotein concentrations.

Dietary fibre is often classified in terms of its solubility. The major insoluble form is cellulose, which represents ß 1-4 linked glucose molecules and represents a major fraction of plant cell wall material. The major soluble fibres are **pectins** and **ß-glucans**. The former are branched polymers of galacturonic acid with other sugars while the latter represent ß1-3 and ß1-4 -linked, branched chains of glucose. The relative amounts of these two types of fibre vary considerably between plant sources. For example in wheat, maize and rice most of the fibre is insoluble while oats and barley contain a significant amount of ß-glucan-rich, soluble fibre. In fruit the relative amounts of soluble and insoluble fibre varies widely with pectin representing the major soluble form.

Most evidence suggests that **insoluble fibre** has little direct effect of lipoprotein metabolism. However, one important effect may simply be the displacement of fat from the diet. Diets rich in fibre tend to be bulky, perhaps increase satiety and as a result lead to reduce consumption of other more energy dense components such as fat and sugar.

By contrast, considerable evidence exists to suggest that **soluble fibre** may have a more direct effect. Numerous animal studies have indicated a cholesterol-lowering effect of either foods rich in soluble fibre or dietary supplements of extracted soluble fibre. There is less direct evidence for such an effect in humans. One meta-analysis, of 10 studies, suggested that an intake of soluble fibre from oats of 3g/day may lower plasma cholesterol by approximately 2% in people with moderate plasma cholesterol levels (5.9mM) and perhaps by more in people with raised levels.

If soluble fibre does decrease plasma cholesterol then what is the mechanism? One possibility is that diets rich in soluble fibre promote the excretion of bile acids perhaps by trapping them in the fibre matrix within the large intestine and preventing their re-absorption. A second proposal has been that fermentation of soluble fibre in the large intestine lead to the production of **short chain fatty acids** that are then absorbed into the body. One such fatty acid, propionate, may directly act by inhibiting cholesterol synthesis in the liver. The relative contribution of these mechanisms to any cholesterol-lowering effects of soluble fibre in humans remains to be established.

8.4 Dietary protein

There is a mass of evidence to suggest that in certain animal species the type and amount of dietary protein can have profound effects on plasma cholesterol concentrations. One of the most sensitive species appears to be the rabbit which, when fed diets containing the milk protein **casein**, develop severe hypercholesterolaemia compared to those fed protein isolated from Soya beans. These observations have also been made in a number of other species although the magnitude of the effect appears to vary considerably. It also appears that differences can be shown between the effects of other animal and plant proteins. These results have led to a number of clinical trials in humans. These studies have produced a wide range of results but in general support a cholesterol-lowering effect of vegetable-protein compared to animal-protein, particularly in people with hypercholesterolaemia. These carefully controlled studies have been able to specifically determine the effect of protein in the absence of changes in the intake of other nutrients. Comparing populations that have large endogenous differences in the source of their dietary protein is much more difficult due to the vast number of differences in dietary intakes of other macro- and micronutrients. How relevant these finding are to the general population is debatable. However, inclusion of vegetable protein (at the expense of animal protein) in the diet of patients with pathologically raised cholesterol levels may represent a useful therapeutic tool.

A number of potential mechanisms have been suggested for the mechanism whereby dietary proteins influence lipoprotein metabolism. One suggestion is that, like dietary fibre, some interaction between an undigested fraction of vegetable protein and bile acids (and perhaps cholesterol itself) leads to an increase in excretion. Others suggest effects are mediated through changes in hormonal status with thyroid hormone, insulin and glucagon all being implicated. In rabbits, the mechanism appears to associated with a modulation of LDL receptor activity and may be associated with specific amino acids within the proteins. Lysine and methionine appear particularly cholesterol raising, while arginine may counteract their effect.

Table 8.2 Recommended macronutrient intakes for reducing cardiovascular disease*

Nutrient	*Current UK intakes (adults 16-64 years)*		*Recommendation*
	Men	*Women*	
Total fat (% total energy)	37.6	39.2	Decrease average to about 35%
Saturated fatty acids (% total energy)	15.4	16.5	Decrease average to about 10%
Monounsaturated fatty acids (% total energy)	11.6	11.8	No recommendation
n-6 polyunsaturated fatty acids (% total energy)	5.1	6.1	No further increase
Long chain n-3 polyunsaturated fatty acids (i.e. EPA & DHA) (g/day)	0.1	0.1	Increase average to about 0.2g/day
Trans -fatty acids (% total energy)	2.0	2.1	Should not increase
Dietary cholesterol (mg/day)	390	280	Should not increase
Dietary carbohydrate (% total energy)	41.6	43.0	Starch & sugars in fruit & vegetables should increase such that total carbohydrate contributes about 50% energy
Dietary fibre	24.9	18.6	No recommendation
Dietary protein (% total energy)	12	12	No recommendation

*Taken from: Department of Health. Report on Health and Social Subjects 46 Nutritional Aspects of Cardiovascular Disease (1994) Report of the Cardiovascular Review Group, Committee on Medical Aspects of Food Policy (London, HMSO)

8.5 Conclusions: dietary recommendations for macronutrient intakes

It is clear from this and the preceding chapter that macronutrient intake can have a major impact on circulating lipoprotein concentrations. The most significant and well-documented effects appear to be those of dietary fats. With the growing awareness that dietary intervention may, through altering lipoprotein concentrations, modulate the risk of developing atherosclerotic disease, numerous attempts have been made to formulate the "ideal" dietary recommendations. The central focus of these has always remained a reduction in the intake of saturated fat. The amount of total, mono- and polyunsaturated fatty acid intake has remained more controversial. Advising bodies have tended to steer away from specific recommendations for carbohydrate, fibre and protein intake. The most recent recommendations from the UK Department of Health (Committee on Medical Aspects of Food Policy) as relating to macronutrients are summarised in table 8.2. While these reflect the current thinking of most countries, individual researchers are beginning to question the wisdom of reducing total fat intake. Thus, two important questions remain to be answered: 1) Are we right to focus on the percentage of fat in the diet or should we be looking at the total amount? 2) What should we replace saturated fatty acids with, carbohydrate or unsaturated fatty acids?

Key references

General

A report of a WHO Study Group. (1990) Diet, nutrition, and the prevention of chronic diseases. World Health Organisation Technical Report Series 797

Report of the panel on dietary reference values of the Committee on Medical Aspects of Food Policy. (1991) Dietary reference values for food energy and nutrients for the United Kingdom. Report on health and social subjects 41. London HMSO

Report of the cardiovascular review group, Committee on Medical Aspects of Food Policy. (1994) Nutritional aspects of cardiovascular disease. Report on health and social subjects 46. London HMSO

Dietary carbohydrates

Truswell, A.S. (1994) Food carbohydrates and plasma lipids - an update. American Journal of Clinical Nutrition, 59, 710S-718S

Frayn, K.N. and Kingman, S.M. (1995) Dietary sugars and lipid metabolism in human. American Journal of Clinical Nutrition, 62, 250S-263S

Dietary fibre

Ripsin, C.M., Keenan, J.M., Jacobs, D.R. *et al*. Oat products and lipid lowering: A meta-analysis. Journal of the American Medical Association 267, 3317-3325

Marlett, J.A. (1997) Sites and mechanisms for the hypocholesterolemic actions of soluble dietary fibre sources In: Dietary Fibre in Health and Disease (Eds D. Kritchevsky and C. Bonfield) Advances in Experimental Medicine and Biology 427 (Plenum Press, New York)

Dietary protein

Carroll, K.K. and Kurowska, E.M. (1995) Soy consumption and cholesterol reduction: review of animal and human studies. Journal of Nutrition 125, 594S-597S

Potter, S.M. (1995) Overview of proposed mechanisms for the hypocholesterolemic effect of soy. Journal of Nutrition 125, 606S-611S

9 Micronutrients

9.1 Introduction

Trace elements and vitamins are known to be required in the diet of man. For example iron is required for haemoglobin biosynthesis and hence is required for the transport of oxygen and thus for respiration. Iron is also present in iron-sulphur proteins and the cytochromes which are essential components of the electron transport chain in mitochondria. Copper is required for the function of the vital terminal constituent of the electron transport chain, cytochrome oxidase and for other important enzymes. Vitamins are required for a wide variety of physiological and biochemical purposes.

Harmful oxidation of structural and functional proteins, lipids and nucleic acids can occur through the action of **free radicals** and **reactive oxygen species** (see below). Certain metals and vitamins, under particular conditions can enhance free radical formation and action and cause oxidative damage: these are then termed **prooxidants**. Generally, however, some of the vitamins have **antioxidant** properties i.e. they prevent the formation of free radicals or they alleviate oxidative damage.

This chapter will consider trace elements and vitamins as prooxidants or antioxidants with particular reference to the oxidation of LDL, as this appears to have a major role in the pathogenesis of atherosclerosis (see chapter 6).

9.2 Free radicals and reactive oxygen species

Free radical formation and reactive oxygen species

A free radical is any chemical species, capable of independent existence, that contains one or more unpaired electrons.

The most reactive free radical known is the **hydroxyl free radical** $^{\bullet}OH$, which can damage almost all biomolecules. Thus hydroxyl radicals, which can be produced by high energy radiation, can cause damage in DNA leading to mutations and cancer. Damage to lipids involves **lipid peroxidation**. The hydroxyl radical attacks and abstracts a proton from a fatty acid side chain in a phospholipid molecule, preferentially from a fatty acid with several double bonds such as arachidonic acid. The hydrogen atoms most readily abstracted are from the bisallylic methylene groups (-CH=CH-**CH_2**-CH=CH-) of polyunsaturated fatty acids.

$$LH + {}^{\bullet}OH \rightarrow L^{\bullet} + H^{\bullet}$$
$$H^{\bullet} + {}^{\bullet}OH \rightarrow H_2O$$

These two reaction result in the destruction of the hydroxyl radical but forms a carbon-centred lipid free radical ($L^{\bullet}$) which may either rearrange to form a conjugated double bond system in the fatty acid side chain or react with molecular oxygen to form a peroxy radical. This subsequently reacts with another fatty acid side chain, abstracting a proton so continuing, or propagating the free radical chain reaction:

$$L^{\bullet} + O_2 \rightarrow LOO^{\bullet}$$
$$LOO^{\bullet} + LH \rightarrow LO_2H + L^{\bullet}$$

One hydroxyl free radical can result in many lipid hydroperoxides which can disrupt membrane function, cause damage to membrane proteins, enzymes or receptors, and can decompose to cytotoxic compounds. Hydroxyl free radicals may be produced *in vivo* by decomposition of peroxynitrite (see chapter 6) or by the reaction of transition metals with H_2O_2.

Another harmful free radical is the **superoxide anion**, $O_2^{\bullet}$. This is a normal metabolite which is either formed accidentally if an electron escapes the electron transport chain in mitochondria and reacts with molecular oxygen:

$$O_2 + e^- \rightarrow O_2^{\bullet}$$

or is produced by certain cells, such as macrophages by the enzyme *NADPH oxidase*. Macrophages produce this free radical as a normal defence mechanism to kill bacteria.

Oxidative damage can be caused by other molecular species, containing oxygen but which are not free radicals. Hence the term **reactive oxygen species** was introduced to encompass hydroxyl, superoxide and nitric oxide radicals along with peroxynitrite, $ONOO^-$, hydrogen peroxide, H_2O_2 and hyperchlorite, HOCl. The latter is secreted by neutrophils as part of the defence against bacterial infection.

Pro-oxidants

Molecules which promote oxidative damage are termed **pro-oxidants**. The transition metals iron and copper are good promoters of free radical reactions as they readily change ionisation state.

$$Fe^{3+} + e^- \rightarrow Fe^{2+}$$
$$Cu^{2+} + e^- \rightarrow Cu^{+}$$

Thus these transition elements can facilitate the following reactions:

$$LOOH + Fe^{2+} \rightarrow LO^{\bullet} + Fe^{3+} + OH^{-}$$
$$LOOH + Fe^{3+} \rightarrow LOO^{\bullet} + Fe^{2+} + H^{+}$$
$$LO^{\bullet} + LH \rightarrow LOH + L^{\bullet}$$
$$LOO^{\bullet} + LH \rightarrow LOOH + L^{\bullet}$$
$$L^{\bullet} + O_2 \rightarrow LOO^{\bullet}$$

Vitamin C, can act as a pro-oxidant under certain circumstances by converting Fe^{3+} to Fe^{2+} and Cu^{2+} to Cu^{+}. The latter and Fe^{2+} react faster with peroxides than the oxidised forms of the metals. Vitamin E can also act as a pro-oxidant, in mild oxidising conditions in the absence of other antioxidants which can convert the tocopherol radical back to the native vitamin form.

9.3 Protection against oxidative damage

Protection can be considered under two headings: primary protection comprising certain enzymes and metal ion sequestration and secondary protection comprising the action of antioxidants.

Primary protection

Various enzymes, often referred to as scavenger enzymes, remove harmful reactive oxygen species. Superoxide radicals may be removed by the enzyme ***superoxide dismutase*** which catalyses the following reaction:

$$O_2^{\bullet} + O_2^{\bullet} + 2H^{+} \rightarrow H_2O_2 + O_2$$

The hydrogen peroxide formed in this reaction and other metabolic routes can be removed either by ***catalase***, reaction (a) below, or by ***glutathione peroxidase***, reaction (b) below. The latter enzyme is interesting as it is the only known enzyme to have a specific requirement for the element **selenium**.

a) $2H_2O_2 \rightarrow 2H_2O + O_2$
b) $2GSH + H_2O_2 \rightarrow GSSG + H_2O$

The enzymes *paroxazone* and *platelet activating factor acyl hydrolase* have a role in the reduction of oxidative damage of LDL. These enzymes are discussed further in chapter 6.

Sequestration of metal ions by storage or transport proteins prevents their participation in oxidative damage. Thus in plasma the protein, **transferrin**, has a binding capacity for iron that is three fold the usual concentration of iron so that free iron is unlikely to occur except under exceptional circumstances. Similarly copper ions are bound to **caeruloplasmin** or **albumin** in plasma and are rarely present in the unbound form.

Secondary protection: antioxidants

Most **free radical trapping antioxidants** stop the propagation of the free radical chain reaction by reacting with a peroxy radical thus:

$$LOO^{\bullet} + AH \rightarrow LOOH + A^{\bullet}$$

The antioxidant radical may wait until it encounters another peroxy radical with which it reacts to give inactive products. The action of certain vitamins as antioxidants is discussed in section 9.4 and their role in protecting LDL from oxidation in section 9.5.

9.4 Antioxidants

In a survey of epidemiological studies, Gey proposed that the data support the hypothesis that sub-optimal levels of principal micronutrients are risk factors for cardiovascular disease. Protective levels of antioxidant vitamins, in plasma, were observed to be >50mM vitamin C, > 30mM lipid standardised vitamin E (α-tocopherol/cholesterol ratio >5.2mmol/mmol) and >0.4mM ß-carotene. The relative risk of symtomatic cardiovascular disease is doubled when these levels are 25-50% lower i.e. sub-optimal. The risk is increased by a sub-optimal level of each vitamin independently and the reduction of two or all three of these vitamins multiplies the risk.

Vitamin E

Vitamin E, in the form of α-tocopherol (see figure 9.1), can act as a free radical chain breaking antioxidant. The tocopheroxyl radical can react with a further alkyl peroxyl radical to yield non radical products or be reduced to the original phenol form by reacting with an aqueous reducing agent such as ascorbic acid (vitamin C; see below). Intracellularly the tocopheroxyl radical can be reduced to tocopherol by reaction with glutathione, catalysed by a membrane specific hydroperoxide glutathione peroxidase which is, as described above, a selenium requiring enzyme. Thus selenium has a direct role in recycling tocopherol inside the cell.

The most common of the 8 naturally occurring homologues, or vitamers, of vitamin E are α-tocopherol and γ-tocopherol (figure 9.1). Different chemical compounds which show the same biological activity are collectively known as vitamers. Tocopherols have saturated side chains,

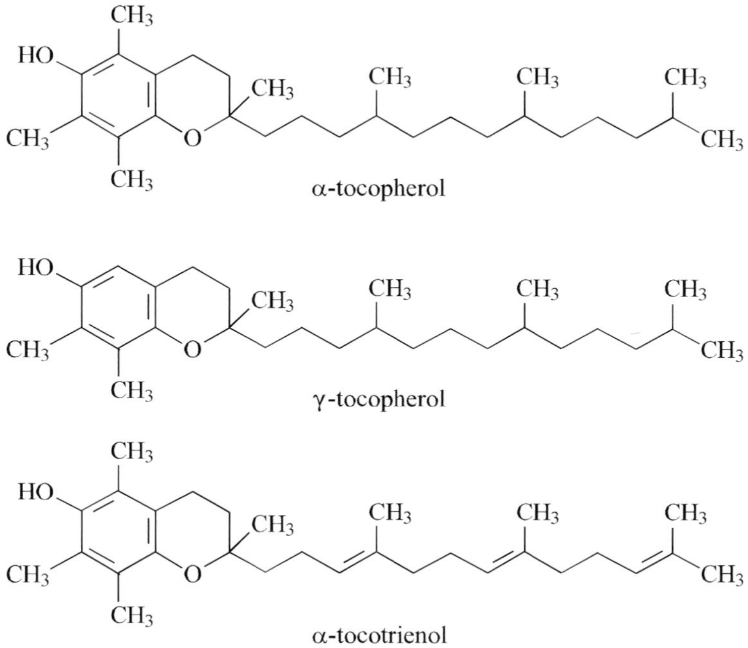

α-tocopherol

γ-tocopherol

α-tocotrienol

Figure 9.1
Vitamin E

tocotrienols have unsaturated side chains. Chemical synthesis yields eight possible stereoisomers of α-tocopherol, some of which have nearly as much biological activity as the natural α-tocopherol. Tocopherols and tocotrienols are important constituents of chloroplast membranes in green plants and are also found in high concentrations in seeds. In man 20-40% of the dietary intake of vitamin E is absorbed, with other dietary lipids. Although the intake of γ-tocopherol may exceed that of α-tocopherol, the γ homologue is usually present in plasma at 10-15% that of the α-tocopherol concentration. Vitamin E is lipid soluble and the various homologues of the vitamin are transported in the blood in the lipoprotein fraction. In plasma, chylomicra contain all forms of tocopherol in the same proportion as the diet whilst VLDL, LDL and HDL contain predominantly the α homologue. This is because the liver contains an α-tocopherol binding (or transfer) protein that promotes the incorporation of a-tocopherol into VLDL : the γ-tocopherol and other vitamers and also excess α-tocopherol are excreted in the bile. Retention of vitamin E in tissues depends upon binding proteins and differs in different tissues: for example the half life of Vitamin E in liver is 9.8 days, in brain 29.4 days and spinal cord 76.3 days.

Deficiency syndromes associated with a lack of vitamin E are rare though they do occur in premature infants or adults with intestinal malabsorption. The reason for the rarity of deficiency is that the vitamin is present in grains, vegetable oils and animal fats, commonly consumed foods. For example the vitamin E content of sunflower oil is 48.7mg/100g, of polyunsaturated margarine 25mg/100g, of hazelnuts 21mg/100g and of wheat germ 11mg/100g. The average vitamin E intake is 8-12mg α-tocopherol per day; in Mediterranean diets the average intake of vitamin E has been estimated at 15mg /day.

Epidemiological studies support a protective role for vitamin E in coronary heart disease. For example the vitamin sub-study of MONICA (monitoring of determinants and trends in cardiovascular disease), in which approximately 100 men, selected at random, from each of 16 countries were studied, found that in the 12 populations with similar cholesterol and blood pressure values there was a significant inverse correlation of vitamin E with the mortality from coronary heart disease. In the whole population studied the four variables, lipid standardised vitamin E, total plasma cholesterol, lipid standardised vitamin A and diastolic blood pressure, predicted the actual coronary heart disease mortality by 87%.

In a four year study, begun in 1986, of 39,910 male health professionals who were initially free from overt coronary heart disease, diabetes and hypercholesterolemia, assessment of dietary vitamin intake revealed a lower risk of subsequent coronary heart disease among men with higher intakes of vitamin E. It was concluded that the data did not prove a causal relation but did provide evidence of an association of a high vitamin E intake with a lower risk of coronary disease in men. Similar effects of vitamin E were found in women in an eight -year study, begun in 1980, of 87,245 nurses, aged between 34 and 59 years and free from overt symptoms of cardiovascular disease at the outset. In both these studies a high intake of vitamin E, usually as a supplement, was associated with a significantly reduced risk of developing coronary heart disease.

The beneficial effect of Vitamin E in protecting against coronary heart disease, is believed to be related to its ability to act as an antioxidant. Thus it is presumed to help protect LDL against oxidative damage by free radicals. The effects of α-tocopherol as an antioxidant in LDL, *in vitro* and *in vivo*, are considered further below (section 9.5). Vitamin E may also have antiatherogenic properties unrelated to its antioxidant capacity. Thus the vitamin has been reported to inhibit smooth muscle cell proliferation *in vitro* and reduces platelet adhesion, properties which should inhibit the progression of atherosclerosis and decrease thrombosis.

Tocotrienols, which are related in structure to a-tocopherol (figure 9.1), reduce plasma cholesterol by acting as HMGCoA reductase inhibitors, i.e. they inhibit endogenous cholesterol biosynthesis. However, as α-

tocopherol reduces this effect, it is uncertain whether the tocotrienols have any significant protective role *in vivo* when conventional diets are consumed.

Vitamin C

Vitamin C, ascorbic acid (figure 9.2), is obtained from fruit and vegetables in the diet. Some 80-95% of dietary ascorbate is absorbed.

Figure 9.2
Vitamin C

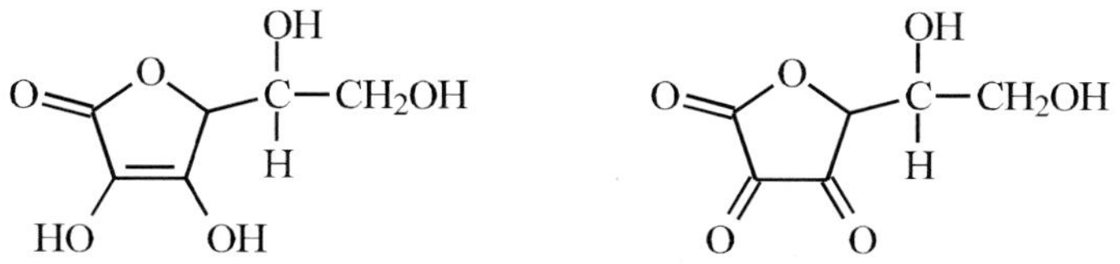

ascorbic acid (vitamin C)

dehydroascorbic acid

Deficiency of the vitamin leads to scurvy in which there are skin lesions and fragile blood vessels. This is because the vitamin is required for hydroxylation of the connective tissue protein, collagen. For example, the enzyme *prolyl hydroxylase* which catalyses hydroxylation of proline residues in collagen thus:

prolyl residue + O_2 + α-ketoglutarate = 4hydroxylprolyl residue + CO_2 + succinate

requires vitamin C to restore the Fe^{2+} in the enzyme. For this purpose the vitamin acts as an antioxidant. It is as an antioxidant that vitamin C may also have an important role in protecting against oxidative damage in atherosclerosis. Vitamin C is also required for other hydroxylation reactions such as those involved in the synthesis of carnitine and noradrenaline and for amidation of certain neuropeptides. Vitamin C is required by *aspartate hydroxylase* which modifies protein kinase C and the vitamin K dependent protease which hydrolyses factor V in the blood clotting cascade.

Plasma ascorbate levels are low in hypertension, in smokers and in myocardial infarction. The low levels may be the result of the disease or an impairment of the recycling mechanism(s) to restore ascorbic acid from dehydroascorbic acid. These mechanisms are not fully understood but may involve non-enzymatic reaction with glutathione, a *dehydroascorbic acid reductase* requiring NADPH and glutathione and an *ascorbyl free radical reductase*.

Dietary supplementation with vitamin C reduced total serum cholesterol and increased HDL in patients with a low vitamin C intake but had little effect upon those whose intake was already adequate. Vitamin C supplementation was thought to be beneficial to health in hypertensive and diabetic patients and in smokers and elderly men, all at increased risk from coronary heart disease.

In the Basle prospective study 2,974 middle aged men were followed for 12 years. In this period there were 132 cases of coronary heart disease and 31 strokes. Plasma antioxidant levels were measured as soon as possible after isolation of plasma. Vitamin E levels were high and mostly above the critical threshold believed to be required for absence of risk of coronary heart disease. Low values of either carotene or vitamin C, or of both, were associated with a moderate but statistically insignificant risk of coronary heart disease. However, the relative risk of cerebrovascular death increased four fold in subjects with low concentrations of both vitamin C and carotene. This result suggests that vitamin C has an important role in protecting against stroke.

The interaction of ascorbate with a-tocopherol in the protection of LDL against oxidation is discussed in section 9.5. below.

Carotenes and vitamin A

Carotenoids, particularly ß-carotene, are the major dietary source of vitamin A (figure 9.3). Carotenoids are a class of hydrocarbons (carotenes) and their oxygenated derivatives (xanthophylls). About 600 carotenoids have been isolated from natural sources: they are found throughout the plant kingdom, giving rise to colour of fruits, bird feathers, insects and marine animals. Animals are unable to synthesise carotenoids.

Vitamin A refers to retinol, its aldehyde retinal and retinoic acid (figure 9.3). However, vitamin A intake usually includes preformed vitamin A, in foods of animal origin, and provitamin carotenoids, in foods of plant origin. Retinol is present in foods mainly as retinol ester, predominantly retinyl palmitate. Some 70-90% of dietary retinol is absorbed from the diet and is transported to the liver in chylomicrons. Retinol is released from the liver bound to retinol binding protein, one mole of retinol per mole of protein. This protein does not bind retinyl palmitate or ß-carotene.

Vitamin A is required for vision: the vitamin is present in opsins which function as signal transducers of light signals received in the retina, transferring the signals to the brain. The vitamin is required for synthesis of some glycoproteins and it functions as a carrier of mannosyl residues. Finally the vitamin is essential for the regulation of growth and development.

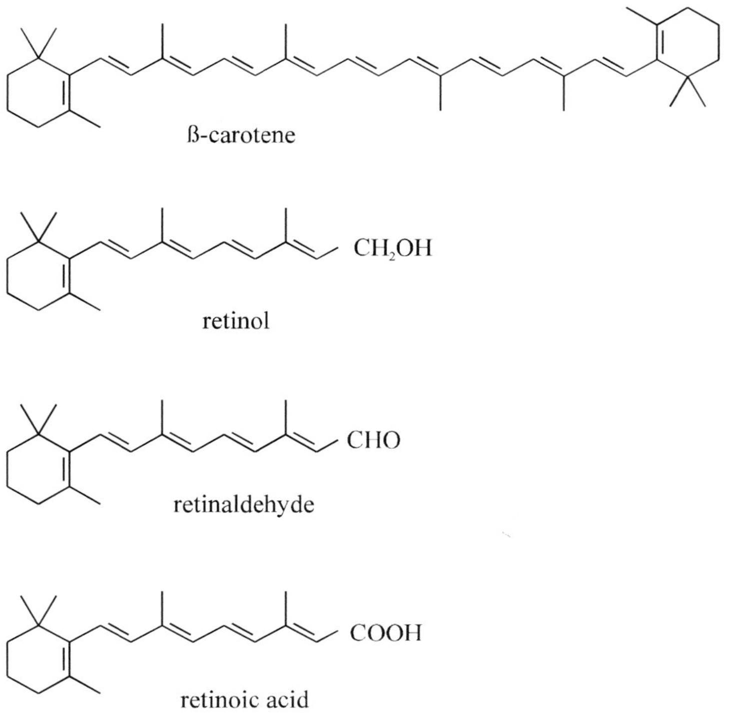

ß-carotene

retinol

CH$_2$OH

Figure 9.3
Carotenoids and vitamin A

retinaldehyde

CHO

retinoic acid

COOH

Deficiency of vitamin A is a major cause of premature death and of blindness in children in certain parts of the world. Care must be taken in treating deficiency, or in supplementing diets with retinol as excess can be toxic.

The carotenoids have extensive conjugated double bonds which gives them potential antioxidant capacity. Despite evidence from *in vitro* studies that carotenoids have antioxidant properties at low oxygen concentrations, it is not clearly established that they have this function *in vivo*. Most epidemiological studies relating to coronary heart disease are of ß-carotene although the carotenoids lycopene and cryptoxanthine may be present in concentrations of similar magnitude to ß-carotene in plasma and plasma retinol concentrations are higher than ß-carotene. The plasma carotenoids, but not retinol, are largely transported in lipoproteins. A low concentration of retinol ester may be associated with LDL.

There is some evidence from ecological, cross-sectional and cohort epidemiological studies that ß-carotene, carotenoids as a group or carotenoid rich foods may have a protective association with coronary heart disease. However, two intervention trials, the Alpha Tocopherol Beta Carotene Study of 29,133 Finnish male smokers and the Beta

Carotene and Retinol Efficacy Trial, of 18314 smokers, former smokers and workers exposed to asbestos showed that supplementation of diets with ß-carotene, 20mg daily, or 30mg ß-carotene with 25,000IU vitamin A daily, respectively, actually increased the risk of heart disease and lung cancer. These results may be related to the harmful effects of free radicals in cigarette smoke or the exposure to asbestos. Alcohol consumption enhanced the risk of development of disease. Supplementation with ß-carotene does not seem to be harmful in apparently healthy people, however. In the Physicians Health Study, of 22,071 male physicians, supplementation was 50mg on alternate days for 12 years and no toxic effects of supplementation was found. In this study only 11% were current smokers but 39% had smoked formerly. No significant effect of ß-carotene supplementation on the risk of cardiovascular disease was obtained in this study .

An association was found between the adipose ß-carotene concentration and myocardial infarction in a case control study of 674 patients and 725 controls in eight European centres and Israel. The strongest association of low ß-carotene concentration with myocardial infarct occurred when the adipose tissue polyunsaturated fatty acid content was high.

Nonetheless, despite equivocal epidemiological data supporting a favourable role of carotenoids and some contraindications for supplementation in the presence of environmental stresses such as asbestos exposure or dietary stress such as smoking or alcoholism, in view of their potentially protective effect on the oxidation of LDL, discussed below, the carotenoids should not be withheld from the diet but consumed in adequate quantity to achieve optimal health. Further research is required to determine the optimal plasma concentration, the extent of absorption, metabolism and bioavailability and function of the individual carotenoids in the diet.

Ubiquinol

Ubiquinol-10 is the reduced form of ubiquinone-10, or coenzyme Q10: the number indicates the number of isoprenyl units in the molecular form commonly found in mammals (see figure 9.4). Ubiqunone is a proton-electron carrier in the inner mitochondrial membrane and is a lipophilic antioxidant in different cell membranes and LDL. Ubiquinol-10 is an endogenous product of the mevalonate pathway and is present in food, particularly soybeans, walnuts, almonds, oils, fruits and spinach.

Flavonoids and polyphenols

Although more than 4,000 different flavonoids have been identified in plant material, few plants have been systematically studied and little is

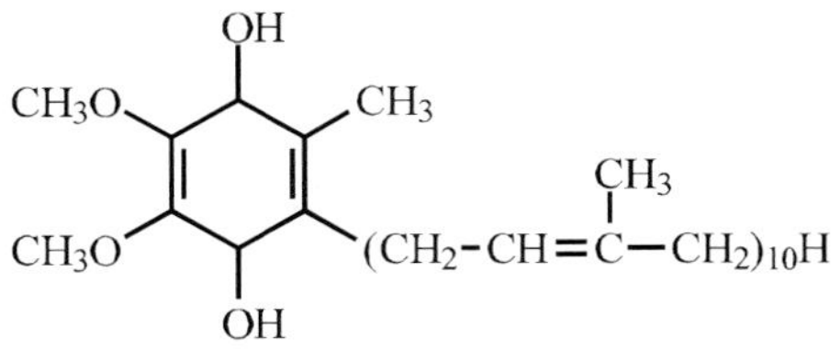

Figure 9.4
Ubiquinol

known about the absorption, bioavailability and metabolism of the more common dietary flavonoids. The major sources of these, in a Western diet, are tea, onions, apples and red wine. The tannins found in tea are polymers of flavonoids. The structure of two commonly ocurring flavonoids found in food are shown in figure 9.5.

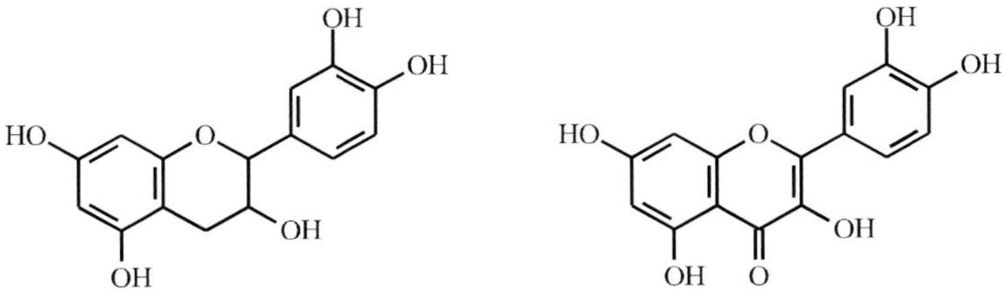

Figure 9.5
Flavonoids: two examples of flavonoids which occur in foods and red wine

(+)-catechin

quercetin

Many flavonoids are antioxidants, free radical scavengers and metal chelators. Examples of these activities *in vitro* have been described. However, the role of flavonoids *in vivo* is unknown. One epidemiological study has investigated the effects of dietary flavonoids: the Zutphen Elderly Study found an inverse association between dietary flavonoid intake and mortality from coronary heart disease. The mean flavonoid consumption was estimated to be 26mg/day with 61% from tea, 13% from onions and 10% from apples. The flavonoid catechin can reduce fatty streak formation in hypercholesterolaemic hamsters and catechin and quercetin were found to reduce the progression of atherosclerosis in apo E deficient mice. In view of the results of these studies, the potential antioxidant capacity of flavonoids and the ability of certain flavonoids to scavenge peroxynitrite and the effect of flavonoids on the oxidation of LDL *in vitro* (see section 9.4), more research is required to determine the role of these compounds in protection against atherosclerosis in humans. Flavonoids may also protect against thrombosis as they can inhibit platelet aggregation.

Paradoxically flavonoids have antitumour activity although the mechanism(s) for the cytotoxic effect on tumour cells is not understood.

The protective effect of red wine and extra virgin olive oil against LDL oxidation (see below) has been attributed to polyphenols. While flavonoids may be classed as polyphenols the chemical nature of the polyphenols in red wine and extra virgin olive oil has not been fully established.

9.5 Oxidation of LDL

Evidence that LDL is oxidised *in vivo* and that oxidised LDL has an important role in the pathogenesis of atherosclerosis is discussed in chapter 6. Some of the studies relating to the effect of various micronutrients on LDL susceptibility to oxidation *in vitro* are discussed below.

LDL oxidation *in vitro*

LDL can be oxidised, *in vitro*, by incubating LDL with cultured endothelial cells, or macrophages or metal ions such as copper or iron, resulting in peroxidation of polyunsaturated fatty acids in the LDL molecule. Formation of lipid peroxides is followed by fragmentation of fatty acids to short chain aldehydes such as malondialdehyde and 4-hydroxynonenal. Some oxidation of cholesterol, within LDL, also occurs. The mechanism(s) of oxidation and the chemical nature of all the oxidation products formed is not fully understood. Oxidation of LDL may be measured in a number of ways but is most readily measured by following the formation of conjugated dienes.

The composition of LDL is shown in table 9.1. LDL usually contains about 6 molecules of α-tocopherol per particle (range 3-9). Some LDL particles also contain a molecule of ubiquinol and/ or a carotenoid molecule. When LDL is oxidised *in vitro* the lag time i.e. the time before fatty acid side chains are oxidised, is dependent upon the total antioxidant content and on the presence of aqueous antioxidants in the immediate vicinity. Ubiquinol can protect LDL from copper induced oxidation and may be the first antioxidant component of LDL to be consumed during oxidation. The oxidizability of LDL *in vitro* correlates negatively with the initial ubiquinol content. Ubiquinol may protect the lipoprotein from lipid peroxidation by scavenging the lipid radicals thus:

$$UQH_2 + LO^\bullet \rightarrow LOH + UQH^\bullet$$
$$UQH_2 + LOO^\bullet \rightarrow LOOH + UQH^\bullet$$

Ubiquinol 10 may protect α-tocopherol thus:

$$UQH_2 + \alpha\text{-}T^\bullet \rightarrow UQH^\bullet + \alpha\text{-}TH$$

Table 9.1 Composition of human LDL (adapted from Esterbauer *et al.*, 1992)

	number of molecules per lipoprotein particle (approximate)
Phospholipid	700
Free cholesterol	600
Cholesterol ester	1600
Triacylglycerol	100
Fatty acid	2700
(polyunsaturated fatty acid)	1300
α-tocopherol	6
γ-tocopherol	0.5
ß-carotene	0.3
Lycopene	0.2

Once ubiquinol and α-tocopherol are utilised then carotenoids become effective antioxidants (see figure 9.6). The ubiquinol and α-tocopherol react more rapidly with peroxyl radicals than polyunsaturated fatty acids and hence act as chain breaking antioxidants. The α-tocopherol radical can be reconverted to a-tocopherol by reaction with ubiquinol, as shown above, or an aqueous antioxidant such as ascorbate (vitamin C). During *in vitro* oxidation of LDL the presence of ascorbate can increase the lag phase.

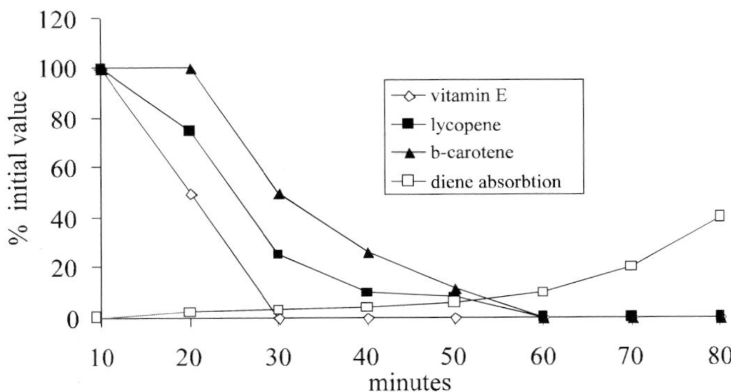

Figure 9.6 Peroxidation of LDL: disappearance of antioxidants and formation of conjugated dienes.

LDL (0.25mg/ml) was incubated in PBS with 1.66μM Cu^{2+}. Absorption was measured at 234 nm. Adapted from Esterbauer *et al.*, 1992

In vitro oxidation of LDL, isolated from normal volunteers, does not appear to correlate with endogenous a-tocopherol concentration. However, it has been found that addition of vitamin E to the plasma before isolation of LDL increases the resistance to oxidation. Several research groups have found that the resistance of isolated LDL to oxidation, *in vitro*, can also be increased by dietary supplementation with vitamin E for some weeks before isolation of LDL. In cell culture studies, intracellular enrichment with vitamin E prevents the oxidative modification of LDL by macrophages. In contrast, the LDL from smokers is more susceptible to oxidation *in vitro* and this may be attributed to the lower content of vitamin E in the LDL.

The α-tocopherol content in LDL in patients with coronary heart disease was found by one group to be lower than that of healthy controls but by another group to be similar to control value. The greater susceptibility to oxidation *in vitro* of LDL from patients with coronary heart disease, in this second study, was attributed to a higher content of polyunsaturated fatty acids in the LDL of these patients. The effect of dietary fat on the oxidation of LDL will be discussed below.

Ascorbate can inhibit the oxidative modification of LDL *in vitro* by a variety of oxidation systems through it's ability to scavenge free radicals and reactive oxygen species and hence preserve the antioxidants present in LDL. The importance of vitamin C, *in vivo*, in relation to the oxidation of LDL is uncertain. The preservation of α-tocopherol and the restoration of α-tocopherol from the radical form may be crucial *in vivo*. Alternatively, the prolongation of the lag phase may protect LDL during its traverse of the sub-endothelial layer of the artery wall to the lymph and to the blood supply and prevent formation of minimally modified and more fully oxidised LDL which can promote foam cell formation and early stages of atherosclerosis.

As only some LDL particles contain carotenoids (see table 9.1) their role in protecting LDL from oxidation is uncertain. Supplementation of the diet with ß-carotene does not affect the oxidation of LDL *in vitro* although this observation does not exclude an antioxidant role for ß-carotene *in vivo*. Plasma carotenoid concentrations are significantly lower in smokers which may contribute, along with a reduced α-tocopherol content, to the greater susceptibility to oxidation of LDL isolated from smokers compared to that from non-smokers.

The flavonoids, +catechin, quercetin and others, inhibit cell induced or copper stimulated LDL oxidation and inhibit the uptake of the oxidised lipoprotein by macrophages. Polyphenols and flavonoids may be responsible for the reduced oxidisability of LDL, in whole plasma resulting from the dietary intake of a South American plant extract known as "Mate". Similarly, consumption of red wine by humans was found to reduce the susceptibility of plasma and LDL to lipid peroxidation and to increase the lag phase of oxidation of LDL. The polyphenol content of LDL was significantly increased by red wine.

The lag time of oxidation of LDL, *in vitro*, was found to be prolonged by a six-month daily supplement of a-tocopherol, vitamin C and ß-carotene. This suggests that the complementary action of these three vitamins may provide protection against the development of atherosclerosis.

As it is the polyunsaturated fatty acids in LDL that are susceptible to peroxidation it was suggested that it might be possible to modify the fatty acid composition of LDL such that it is less susceptible to oxidation. LDL isolated from subjects on an oleate-enriched diet was compared to LDL isolated from subjects on a linoleate-rich diet. The former contained more oleate and less linoleate than the latter and was less susceptible to oxidation. Within the LDL fraction there are particles differing in density. The less dense particles are less susceptible to oxidation than the more dense particles. The former contains more α-tocopherol and a higher ratio of oleate to linoleate. Dietary supplementation with olive oil (rich in oleate and various antioxidants) decreases the susceptibility of LDL to *in vitro* oxidation, decreases the uptake of isolated LDL by macrophages and also decreases the content of cholesteryl ester and increases the free cholesterol content of the LDL.

LDL oxidation *in vivo*

In vivo, LDL oxidation in the blood is prevented by α-tocopherol and other antioxidants within the LDL particle, by vitamin C and other water -soluble antioxidants such as flavonoids and by albumin and HDL. Only traces of oxidised LDL are present in the blood stream and it is possible that these are from efflux from atherosclerotic regions of the artery wall. Once in the sub-endothelial region of the artery wall the LDL particles may be bound by matrix components and become separated from protective albumin and HDL particles, and if lipid soluble and aqueous antioxidants are low in concentration, the lipids of the LDL particle may be exposed to free radicals and lipid peroxidation may ensue. The results of the studies described above suggest that LDL oxidation may be prevented by an adequate supply of antioxidant molecules within LDL and in the sub-endothelial space. Conversely, in the presence of suboptimal levels of antioxidants, peroxidation of LDL would be more likely to occur and the damage that oxidised LDL can produce (see chapter 6) would be unimpeded, causing the development of atherosclerosis.

9.6 Conclusion

Certain metals and vitamins can, under certain circumstances, act as pro-oxidants. Whether they act in this fashion, or act as antioxidants, *in vivo*, is uncertain. However the beneficial effect of diets rich in fruit and vegetables, which are likely to be high in content of the major antioxidant vitamins, would suggest that these vitamins do indeed have a major role as antioxidants, *in vivo*. Therefore, in view of the potential role of oxidised LDL in the pathogenesis of atherosclerosis, diets rich in fruit and vegetables should be recommended for the prevention of atherosclerosis.

As vitamin E is present mainly in vegetable oils and animal fats it may be difficult to increase the intake of this vitamin without increasing the fat content of the diet. An alternative, if the vitamin E content of the diet is low, would be to recommend vitamin E supplements. However the efficacy of vitamin E remains to be fully established. The antioxidant capacity of the diet in general is still not fully understood as some of the plant polyphenols may act in a similar fashion to vitamin C and act to extend the antioxidant capacity of vitamin E.

Key references

General

Trace elements in human nutrition and health (1996) WHO

Bender, D.A. (1992) Nutritional biochemistry of the vitamins. Cambridge University Press

Halliwell, B. (1989) Current status review: free radicals, reactive oxygen species and human disease with special reference to atherosclerosis. British Journal Experimental Pathology. 70, 737-757

Gey, K.F. (1995) Ten year retrospective on the antioxidant hypothesis of arteriosclerosis: threshold plasma levels of antioxidant micronutrients related to minimum cardiovascular risk. Journal of Nutritional Biochemistry 6, 206-236

Vitamin E

Gey, K.F. *et al*. (1991) Inverse correlation between vitamin E and mortality from ischemic heart disease in cross cultural epidemiology. American Journal Clinical Nutrition 53 326S-334S

Dutta-Roy, A.K. *et al*. (1994) Vitamin E requirements, transport and metabolism: role of a tocopherol binding proteins. Journal Nutritional Biochemistry 5, 562-570

Stamfer, M.J. and Rimm, E.B. (1995) Epidemiological evidence for vitamin E in the prevention of cardiovascular disease. American Journal Clinical Nutrition 62, 1365S-1369S

Vitamin C

Levine, M. *et al*. (1996) Vitamin C pharmokinetics in healthy volunteers: evidence for a recommended dietary allowance. Proceedings of the National Academy of Science 93, 3704-3709

Bode, A.M. (1997) Metabolism of vitamin C in health and disease. Advances of Pharmacology 38, 21-47

Carotenoids and Vitamin A

Pfander, H. (1992) Carotenoids: an overview. Methods in Enzymology 213, 3-13

Kohlmeier, L. and Hastings, S. (1995) Epidemiological evidence of a role of carotenoids in cardiovascular disease prevention. American Journal Clinical Nutrition 62, 1370S-1376S

G.S.Omenn, G.S. *et al*. (1996) Effects of a combination of beta carotene and vitamin A on lung cancer and cardiovascular disease. New England Journal of Medicine 334, 1150-1155

Ubiquinol

Kontush, A. *et al*. (1995) Antioxidant activity of ubiquinol-10 at physiologic concentrations in human low density lipoprotein. Biochimica Biophysica Acta. 1258, 177-187

Flavonoids

Cook, N. and Sammon (1996)Flavonoids- chemistry, metabolism, cardioprotective effects and dietary sources. Journal of Nutritional Biochemistry 7, 66-76

Aviram, M. and Fuhrman, B. (1998) Polyphenolic flavonoids inhibit macrophage-mediated oxidation of LDL and attenuate atherogenesis. Atherosclerosis 137, S45-S50

LDL oxidation

Esterbauer, H. *et al*. (1992) Biochemical, structural and functional properties of oxidised low density lipoprotein. Frontiers in Molecular Toxicology, 247-262

Esterbauer, H., Schmidt, R. and Hayn,M. (1997) Relationships among oxidation of low density lipoprotein, antioxidant protection and atherosclerosis. Advances in Pharmacology 38, 425-455

10 Obesity, Diabetes and Atherosclerosis

10.1 Introduction

Obesity and diabetes are two metabolic syndromes which are increasing in prevalence in the Western World and which are increasing the burden on the Health Service in the UK and other countries. Both are associated with considerable increases in risk of developing coronary heart disease (CHD). We have all used the subjective sentence "I am fat" or "he is fat", and most of us know that the word obese means grossly fat or grossly overweight. So what causes someone to become overweight and what constitutes obesity? What is the evidence that excess fat is harmful and should obesity be avoided? How is obesity, a disorder of lipid metabolism, related to diabetes, a disorder of carbohydrate metabolism? Some of these questions will be answered below.

10.2 Obesity

Obesity comprises a heterogeneous group of disorders in which body weight is greatly increased. Over 75% of the increase in weight is due to an increase in body fat in the adipose tissues. There is also a lesser increase in non-fat mass. There are a number of ways of classifying obesities. Broadly they may be divided into two groups: those in which the number of fat cells, or **adipocytes**, is increased (hyperplastic or hypercellular adiposity) or those in which the adipocytes are grossly enlarged in size (hypertrophic adiposity). Generally, though not exclusively, the obesity seen in children is of the former type and adult onset obesity is of the latter type. As it is not easy to measure adipose cell size and number, other methods of classification have been used. A person's weight usually correlates with the amount of body fat. **Body mass index** (**BMI**: ratio of weight to the square of the height, kg/m^2), is often used as a measure of obesity (table 10.1). Although the BMI does not distinguish between excess fat and excess muscle weight, and there may be variation between distribution of adiposity between people with the same BMI, it has been a useful general measure of obesity for epidemiological studies.

Epidemiological studies have shown that there is an increased risk of early mortality in the obese compared with people of normal weight and a significantly increased risk of developing cardiovascular disease. The Framingham Study found an increased predisposition for coronary heart disease in the overweight (see chapter 3). In the Nurses Health Study, in which the health and mortality of 115,195 registered nurses in US was followed for sixteen years, it was found that there was a five-fold increase in risk of death from CHD in subjects with a BMI of $> 30 kg/m^2$

Table 10.1 Classification of Obesity by Body Mass Index[1]

BMI	Grade	Description
<20	-	Underweight
20-24.9	0	Desirable range
25-29.9	I	Overweight
30-40	II	Obese
>40	III	Very Obese

compared with women of BMI < 19 kg/m^2. Even moderate gains in weight during adult life can increase the risk of coronary heart disease in middle aged women. The women with the lowest risk were those who were lean at eighteen years of age and did not gain or lose weight after this time. In those who did gain weight after the age of eighteen, there was a 3.1% increase in risk for each kg weight gained.

Men may have an even greater increased risk of developing cardiovascular disease when obese. Examination of the distribution of increased adipose mass by such measurements as waist/hip ratio and comparing the risk of developing cardiovascular disease of different distributions of increased adipose mass has shown that there is more risk attached to increased upper body fat (also termed android, truncal or visceral fat) than lower body fat (also termed gynoid or gluteal fat). The former is more common in men.

The overall cause of obesity is relatively simple; the intake of energy exceeds energy expenditure. Both genetic and environmental factors play an important part in the aetiology of obesity. Obesity can also accompany endocrine imbalance or treatment with certain drugs. Various types of obesity are summarised in table 10.2. The present discussion will be confined to the dietary induced obesities.

The reason why some people get fat has been the subject of intense research for many years. Many obese people claim to eat no more than their non-obese peers but still put on weight. This would suggest some impairment of energy expenditure rather than intake. However, for the vast majority of obese subjects it appears that the primary cause is an over consumption of calories during the active accumulation of fat tissue. This may be exacerbated by a low level of physical activity but there is little evidence for major differences in metabolic rate. So the next question must be, why do some people over-eat? Much research has also gone into the effect of dietary composition and obesity. A number of researchers have maintained that diets rich in fat may be more likely to lead to obesity than those, of an equivalent energy content, rich in carbohydrate. However, as yet, there is little direct evidence that this is the case. High fat, energy dense, diets may lead to energy over-consumption due to effects of satiety (feeling full).

Table 10.2
Types of obesity

Type of obesity	Associated with:	Further characterisation
Diet induced	Nutritional imbalance: high fat, high calorie diet Cafeteria diets	Chronic over-eating in the genetically susceptible
Physical inactivity	Enforced post-operative Ageing	
Drug induced	Corticosteroids Psychotropic drugs	
Neuroendocrine obesities	Hypothalamic syndrome	Malignancy, surgery, trauma, inflammatory disease involving ventro-medial region of hypo-thalamus
	Cushings disease Hypothyroidism Polycystic ovarian syndrome	
	Hypogonadism	Hypofunction of gonads, hyperfunction of pituitary adrenal system and hyperphagia (overeating)
	Growth hormone deficiency Insulinoma	

Genetic factors are involved in the development of obesity. Family studies show a correlation of body weight between parents and children and between siblings. There is a high correlation between body weight of monozygous twins and pairs of twins tend to accumulate fat and fat free mass in a similar manner. Various genes have been linked with obesity in animal models. A major breakthrough was made in 1994 with the discovery of the hormone, **leptin**. Leptin is produced by adipose tissue and interacts with receptors in a number of sites in the body, including the hypothalamus. Through it's interaction with the hypothalamus leptin may play a role in regulating satiety, and hence food intake. The importance of leptin is most clearly seen in the ob/ob mouse. These mutant animals are unable to produce leptin and as a result eat in an uncontrolled way and become grossly obese. A similar pattern emerges in the db/db mouse in which it is not the production of leptin that is affected but the action of the leptin receptor. This has led to intense research into the role of leptin in human obesity. It appears that, in some vary rare cases, human obesity may be associated with leptin deficiency. However, in most obese humans leptin levels are normal or even high. This suggest that insensitivity to the actions of leptin may be a more important factor in the aetiology of human obesity.

The number of obese in different populations varies widely: two extremes and the approximate values for the UK are shown in table 10.3. The prevalence of obesity depends upon sex, race, age and socioeconomic circumstances. Various social factors may lead to overeating, such as frequent business lunches, increased availability of food, the pressure of advertising and high calorie snack food. The level of obesity in the US and the UK appears to be increasing steadily so that it is becoming more of a financial concern as the related medical problems associated with this disorder increase.

Table 10.3 Obesity rates in different parts of the world

Country (date of report of data)	*Percentage of population with BMI > 30kg/m²*	
	Men	*Women*
China (rural)(1992)	1.4	3.1
UK (1993)	13	16
Polynesia (urban) (1991)	58.4	76.8

Obesity is usually accompanied by **insulin resistance** and hyperlipidaemia. A proportion of obese people develop diabetes and many obese people suffer from cardiovascular disease. These complications of obesity are discussed below.

Action of Insulin

Normal action

The primary function of insulin is often regarded as the regulation of glucose homeostasis. However, it also plays important roles in both lipid and protein metabolism. The major effects of insulin are summarised in table 10.4.

Insulin stimulates glucose transport into muscle and adipose cells, by stimulating the translocation of glucose transporters to the cell membrane, increases glycogen synthesis in adipose, muscle and liver, stimulates glucose oxidation by increasing the activity of *pyruvate dehydrogenase* and reduces hepatic output of glucose by inhibiting gluconeogenesis. These actions of insulin are summarized in table 10.4. Insulin stimulates lipogenesis in adipose and liver, by increasing the uptake of glucose and activity of *acetyl CoA carboxylase* and *pyruvate dehydrogenase*, increases the synthesis of triacylglycerol by increasing glycerophosphate concentration and inhibits lipolysis in adipose tissue.

Table 10.4
Effects of Insulin

Metabolic pathway affected	*Insulin promotes:*	*Mode of action at molecular level*
Carbohydrate Metabolism	Increased glucose transport into muscle and adipose tissue	Stimulation of the translocation of glucose transporters to the cell membrane
	Increased glycogen synthesis in muscle and liver	Activation of glycogen synthase by inhibition of glycogen synthase kinase-3
	Inhibition of glucone-ogenesis	Inhibition of trans-cription of phosphoenol pyruvate carboxykinase
	Glycosaminoglycan biosynthesis	
Lipid Metabolism	Increased lipogenesis in adipose tissue and muscle	Activates acetyl CoA carboxylase and pyruvate dehydrogenase
	Decreased lipolysis	Inhibits the hormone sensitive lipase of adi-pose tissue by activating phosphodiesterase which reduces cAMP concentrations
	Decreased VLDL secretion	Increased apoB degradation
Protein Metabolism	Amino acid transport (all cells) Protein biosynthesis (all cells). Increased initiation of translation	Phosphorylation of binding protein leads to increased amount of e1F-4E able to form complexes
	Protein catabolism	
Electrolyte Physiology	Stimulation of ATP dependent Na^+/K^+ pump	

Lipolysis of triacylglycerol by the enzyme ***hormone sensitive lipase*** is inhibited by insulin through the activation of a *phosphodiesterase* which reduces cyclic AMP concentration. VLDL secretion from liver is also inhibited by the hormone as insulin increases the degradation of apoB. Insulin reduces ketogenesis via it's activation of *pyruvate dehydrogenase* in liver.

Insulin also promotes protein anabolism, by stimulating amino acid uptake into cells, stimulating the initiation of translation and stimulating the transcription of some genes. Insulin stimulates the ATP dependent Na^+/K^+ pump in all cells. Some of the effects of insulin are seen within a few minutes (acute effects) whilst others take some hours to occur (chronic effects).

It can be seen from the above that insulin has an important role in the regulation of metabolism in the adipose tissue. Thus, the hormone stimulates glucose uptake and glucose oxidation, stimulates lipogenesis and stimulates triacylglycerol biosynthesis in this tissue. Conversely, insulin inhibits intracellular lipolysis. Insulin also activates other enzymes involved in fatty acid uptake by the adipose by inducing the expression of **peroxisome proliferator-activated receptor (PPARγ)**. This is a nuclear transcription factor which, after forming a heterodimer with retinoid X receptor (receptor for 9-*cis*-retinoic acid), binds to DNA and increases the transcription *of lipoprotein lipase (LPL), acylCoA synthetase*, aP2 and a number of other enzymes involved in fatty acid metabolism.

TAG biosynthesis in adipose is stimulated by insulin and also by the **Acyl Stimulatory Protein (ASP)**. This protein acts synergistically to insulin. ASP binds to a specific membrane receptor and acts via a *protein kinase* C signal transduction pathway to increase glucose uptake and to stimulate *diacylglycerol acyl transferase*, the last enzyme in TAG biosynthesis.

Insulin has important effects on many aspects of metabolism and cell growth. These effects are the result of the binding of insulin to it's receptor, the activation of the insulin receptor *tyrosine kinase* and the stimulation of various signal transduction pathways.

Insulin activation of *phosphatidyl inositol 3-kinase* may promote translocation of the enzyme. This has been shown to accompany the relocation of glucose transporters to the cell membrane and may also be involved in the increased degradation of apoB promoted by insulin. In the latter case the *phosphatidyl inositol 3-kinase* is translocated to the endoplasmic reticulum, where apoB synthesis and degradation occurs.

Insulin resistance

Insulin resistance has been defined as the state (of a cell, tissue, system or body) in which a greater than normal amount of insulin is required to produce a quantitatively normal response. It occurs in obesity, diabetes and in certain other conditions such as polycystic ovarian syndrome. Although mutations of the insulin receptor are known, these account for only a few cases of insulin resistance. There is evidence that the defect(s) lies in the post receptor signal transduction pathway in the insulin resistance of obesity. One possible molecular defect which could account for insulin resistance is an increased activity of the protein-***tyrosine phosphatase*** which attenuates the autophosphorylation of the insulin receptor. Such an increase has been reported in the adipose and muscle of obese subjects.

It has been suggested that insulin resistance is the primary cause of **syndrome X**, or the **metabolic syndrome**, a syndrome in which insulin resistance, obesity, hypertension, hyperlipidaemia and diabetes are the symptoms. However, each of these conditions can occur independently and each may be a polygenic disease.

Obesity and Atherosclerosis

The extra weight carried by an obese person puts an extra load on the heart. This organ becomes enlarged and stroke and blood volume increase to meet the additional demand of increased body mass. It is not surprising therefore that obesity is associated with hypertension. Part of the increased susceptibility to cardiovascular disease, seen in the obese, may be due to the hypertension and part may be due to the altered lipoprotein profile.

How does this altered lipoprotein profile arise? An increased production of VLDL results from an increase in delivery of fatty acids to the liver. Free fatty acids enter the capillaries within adipose tissue from the activity of the two lipases; hormone sensitive lipase hydrolyses intracellular TAG and LPL hydrolyses TAG in lipoproteins in the capillaries. Intracellular lipolysis is inhibited indirectly by insulin, as described above, and activated by catecholamines and glucocorticoids. Shortly after a meal, when glucose stimulates the release of insulin from the pancreas, the concentration of plasma free fatty acids fall. Conversely as insulin levels fall the fatty acid concentration rises to an average value of about 0.5mM. Higher concentrations occur during starvation, during exercise or during insulin resistance. The half life of plasma fatty acids is 3-4min. Free fatty acids are a major fuel in human metabolism and their oxidation, and the associated release of energy, is of particular importance in skeletal muscle, heart, kidney and liver. In the latter organ, fatty acids are also incorporated into TAG and either stored in lipid droplets or assembled into VLDL.

Normally about half of the fatty acids released from chylomicrons or VLDL by LPL are removed by the adipose and the remainder enter the general circulation to be taken up by muscle and the liver. If the uptake of fatty acids by the adipose tissue is reduced by insulin resistance or reduction of the ASP pathway, more fatty acids enter the circulation.

These, along with fatty acids released from adipose tissue by the action of hormone sensitive lipase which is no longer supressed by insulin, will increasingly compete with glucose for oxidation by muscle, thereby promoting hyperglycaemia, and will increase VLDL synthesis by the liver. If insulin activity in the liver is also impaired then apoB degradation is reduced enabling more VLDL to be secreted, thereby promoting hyperlipoproteinaemia.

The uptake of fatty acids by adipose tissue has been referred to as fatty acid trapping (as the fatty acids are trapped as acylCoA derivatives first and then as TAG). It may seem paradoxical that reduced fatty acid trapping may be the defect in the obese who store more TAG in the adipose tissue than their lean counterparts. However the reduction of fatty acid uptake by adipose from chylomicrons results in an increase in plasma free fatty acids and increased VLDL biosynthesis by the liver. If more of these lipoprotein particles reach the adipose tissue compared with a normal individual, more fatty acids may be removed from the latter lipoprotein so that the net uptake per day by the adipose may be greater. Defective fatty acid trapping may be an important mechanism in promoting atherogenic dyslipoproteinaemia. An alternative, or perhaps additional mechanism of the production of an atherogenic lipoprotein profile in obesity, is the enhanced regulation of metabolism by the hormones antagonistic to insulin, particularly glucocorticoids, in the presence of insulin resistance.

In the obese the increased VLDL production and reduced LPL activity, leads to hypertriglyceridaemia and increased VLDL remnants, and these along with the reduced HDL production promote atherosclerosis and consequent cardiovascular disease. The reduction in HDL may be due to the failure of insulin to stimulate PPARα, the liver form of the peroxisome proliferator activated receptor. Activation of PPARα stimulates transcription of apoAI and apoAII, the apolipoproteins found in HDL.

Clinically significant coronary lesions are associated with abdominal obesity. From studies of autopsies of young men, without evidence of cardiovascular disease before death, it was found that the severity of clinically silent lesions in atherosclerosis- prone regions of the coronary arteries was also associated with abdominal fatness as measured by the waist/hip ratio. These results show the importance of preventing weight gain to prevent the progression of clinically silent lesions to clinically overt lesions leading to myocardial infarct.

10.3 Diabetes

Diabetes comprises a group of metabolic disorders of glucose metabolism in which glucose is not utilised properly and accumulates in the blood. The cause is a lack of function of insulin, either through an absence of the hormone or a relative resistance to available hormone. Insulin, which is synthesised in and secreted from the beta-cells of the islets of Langerhans in the pancreas, has, as described above, a profound effect upon the metabolism of carbohydrates, lipids, proteins and upon electrolyte balance. Thus a reduction in activity of this important hormone results in profound disruption of biochemical and physiological homeostasis. The two major forms of diabetes are described below. These and secondary forms of diabetes associated with other conditions are summarised in table 10.5.

Table 10.5 Different forms of Diabetes

Diabetes Mellitus	
Primary	Insulin Dependent Diabetes Mellitus (IDDM) (Type I)
	Non Insulin Dependent Diabetes Mellitus (NIDDM) (Type II)
Secondary	Pancreatic disease; Pancreatitis, Haemochromatosis, Neoplastic disease, pancreatectomy
	Liver disease
	Over production or activity of antagonistic hormones; Acromegaly (growth hormone)
	Cushing's syndrome (glucocorticoids)
	Hyperthyroidism (thyroid hormone)
	phaechromocytoma (catecholamines)
	glucagonoma (glucagon)
	pregnancy (human placental lactogen)
	Drug induced; corticosteroids thiazide diuretics

The main biochemical feature characteristic of diabetes is hyperglycaemia, an increased concentration of glucose in the blood. Diabetes has been defined as present if the fasting concentration of glucose in venous plasma is above 7.8 mM (6.7mM in whole blood) and above 11.1 mM (10.0 mM) two hours after an oral glucose dose of 75g. However a recent recommendation by the American Diabetes Association has proposed a diagnosis of diabetes when the fasting plasma glucose is above 7.0 mM.

The incidence of diabetes in Britain is between 1 and 2% of the population and appears to be increasing. The incidence in those of the population of Asian descent is significantly higher. Diabetics are prone to develop one or more of the chronic disorders associated with the disease: diabetic retinopathy, diabetic neuropathy, diabetic nephropathy and atherosclerosis. The pathological changes of atherosclerosis in the diabetic are similar to those in the nondiabetic person but occur earlier and are more severe. About 70% of deaths in diabetics are attributable to atherosclerosis.

Insulin Dependent Diabetes Mellitus (IDDM)

This form of diabetes accounts for only 5-10% of diabetics and usually begins in childhood. IDDM, which appears to be a slow autoimmune disease, progresses over a number of years and it is not until over 90% of the beta-cells of the pancreas are destroyed that the clinical symptoms appear. The clinical symptoms, described below, manifest themselves abruptly and must be treated promptly as some of these patients may present with ketoacidosis which, if untreated, can be fatal. The patient with IDDM is dependent upon daily administration of insulin to sustain life.

The susceptibility to IDDM is directly related to the Human Leucocyte Antigens (HLA), part of the cluster of genes on chromosome 6 known as the Major Histocompatability Complex.These proteins are found on the surface of antigen presenting cells and present peptides to T cell receptors. Polymorphisms of HLA have been identified which are associated with the disease. However, this defect is not sufficient on its own for development of IDDM and environmental factors also appear to be involved. Animal studies suggest that viral infection (with rubella or coxsackie virus) or toxic chemicals could be involved. Congenital rubella infection has been linked to the development of IDDM in humans. New cases of IDDM have antibodies to islet cells in their blood and mononuclear cell infiltration of islet cells and selective destruction of these cells has been observed. The presence of two or more autoantibodies to islet cells can be used to diagnose pre-diabetes in children and in relatives of patients with IDDM.

Lack of insulin in IDDM

The clinical symptoms of IDDM are due to lack of insulin. There is a marked increase in glucose concentration in the blood (hyperglycaemia) and if the renal threshold for the reabsorption for glucose is exceeded glucose will be present in the urine (glucosuria). There is a reduced rate of water reabsorption in the kidney so that excessive urine excretion (polyuria) occurs and this is accompanied by an excessive thirst. A rapid loss of weight and muscle wasting is observed due to increased lipolysis in adipose and increased protein catabolism in muscle. Insulin can acutely enhance sodium reabsorption in the kidney so that in its absence more sodium is excreted. Salt and water loss can lead to tachycardia and hypotension. Ketogenesis is increased and the increase in ketone bodies in the blood (ketonaemia) may lead to increased ketones in the urine (ketonuria) and acetone smell in the breath. The presence of ketonaemia and ketonuria is referred to as ketosis. The increased free fatty acids and ketone bodies in the blood lead to an acidosis (often termed ketoacidosis), that can cause coma and death if not treated.

Non Insulin Dependent Diabetes Mellitus (NIDDM)

NIDDM accounts for as many as 90% of the cases of diabetes encountered. The vast majority of people developing this disease are obese and middle-aged. The symptoms, which are less severe at the outset than IDDM, are caused by an impaired response to insulin. As already described, insulin resistance is often associated with obesity. However, in most cases this is overcome by the production of more insulin by the pancreas and in obese people plasma insulin levels often increase more than in non-obese people in response to dietary carbohydrate. NIDDM appears to occur when, due to some genetic predisposition, the pancreas loses its ability to maintain this high rate of insulin secretion. Thus, for symptoms of diabetes to appear both insulin resistance (discussed above) and defective secretion of insulin are necessary. These patients are not usually responsive to exogenous insulin but require some other medication to reduce the hyperglycaemia. Some of the hypoglycaemic drugs used in the treatment of NIDDM are described below.

The genetic factors underlying most NIDDM have not been identified but a mutation of the *glucokinase* gene is responsible for some of the cases of Maturity Onset Diabetes in the Young (MODY), a rare form of NIDDM. Genetic defect(s) are involved in the development of NIDDM as people with close relatives with the disease are more at risk of developing diabetes of this form.The incidence of NIDDM is particularly high in the Pima Indians in Arizona (35%). Hyperinsulinaemia is an early abnormality seen in those, of this race, who subsequently develop NIDDM. Those who do develop NIDDM also develop defective insulin secretion. Further support for a polygenic basis for many cases of NIDDM, is given by the studies on transgenic knockout mice. Neither the insulin receptor substrate deficient mice, that have normal glucose tolerance despite insulin resistance, nor the pancreatic *glucokinase* deficient mice, which have reduced glucose tolerance due to decreased insulin secretion in response to elevated glucose, have symptoms of diabetes. However the mice obtained from crossing these two knockout strains, which are deficient in both genes, develop overt diabetes.

Many of people with NIDDM are obese (> 80%) but not all obese people have diabetes. Hence obesity may predispose someone who has the genetic susceptibility for diabetes to develop the disease. NIDDM usually presents in middle age. By the time the symptoms are recognised as diabetes, some of the patients will have already developed diabetic complications.

Insulin resistance in NIDDM

Only a small percentage of insulin resistant subjects have defective insulin receptors and only a few molecular defects of the glucose transporter have been described. Kinetic studies in NIDDM and lean non-diabetic subjects showed that the defect in insulin resistance is in one or more post-insulin receptor component of the signal transduction mechanism.

As mentioned above, insulin resistance must also be accompanied by defective insulin secretion for the development of NIDDM. In the healthy person, high blood glucose levels, such as occur after a meal, stimulate the secretion of insulin from the pancreas to deal with the hyperglycaemia. This compensatory mechanism must be lost in NIDDM for hyperglycaemia produced by insulin resistance to be prolonged and symptoms of diabetes to prevail.

Diabetic complications

Diabetes is frequently accompanied by disorders of the vasculature. These may be microvascular, affecting mainly capillaries (termed **diabetic microangiopathy**), or macrovascular, affecting the large blood vessels. The former may affect the eye (**diabetic retinopathy**), the kidney (**diabetic nephropathy**) or the nervous system (**diabetic neuropathy**). Peripheral vascular disease and/ or neuropathy may produce the classic symptom of poorly treated diabetes- the diabetic foot. Microvascular disease appears to be directly related to the control of blood glucose. Thus, the patient who can maintain prevailing blood glucose concentrations as close as possible to normal may prevent, or at least delay, the onset of these debilitating conditions. Macrovascular disease is specifically related to an increased susceptibility to atherosclerosis. While blood glucose control may related to this it appears that even the "well-controlled" diabetic is at increased risk.

Diabetes and Atherosclerosis

The risk factors for developing the clinical symptoms of atherosclerotic disease are the same in diabetics as in the general population. In a prospective study involving twenty three medical centres, and clinical data from 2693 patients with NIDDM, five potentially modifiable risk factors were identified: increased concentration of LDL cholesterol, decreased concentration of HDL cholesterol, raised blood pressure, hyperglycaemia and smoking. This study also confirmed earlier findings that patients with NIDDM have an increased mortality from coronary artery disease compared with the general population.

Many diabetics develop hyperlipoproteinaemia. This may be due to the insulin resistance so that increased synthesis of VLDL occurs and inhibition of apoB secretion by insulin is removed so that VLDL secretion from liver is increased. The diabetic hyperlipoproteinaemia is frequently of typeIV or V, characterised by increased plasma VLDL and sometimes chylomicrons.

The reason that diabetics are more susceptible to developing atherosclerosis is the presence of a more atherogenic lipoprotein profile and may also be related to one or more of the abnormalities found in the endothelium or extracellular matrix of the arterial intima. A reduction in heparin sulphate in the intima may alter the permeability properties, alter the retention time of LDL, and modify the coagulation properties of the vessel wall. Each of these properties may also be affected by non-enzymic glycation of extracellular matrix proteins or proteins of cell membranes, including cell receptors. Non-enzymatically modified proteins and lipids known as advanced glycosylation end products are found localised in atherosclerotic lesions in diabetics. Glycation of LDL itself has been shown to increase the susceptibility of the lipoprotein to oxidation *in vitro* and oxidised glycated LDL (glyc.oxLDL) impairs endothelial function to a greater extent than oxidised LDL. This latter effect of glyc.oxLDL may be due to a stimulation of superoxide production, which reduces the effective concentration and thus the action of nitric oxide (see chapter 6).

The susceptibility of LDL to oxidation in diabetes may depend upon the nutritional status and metabolic control level in each particular subject. Thus LDL from subjects with poor nutrition and poor treatment of their diabetes may be much more susceptible to oxidation than LDL from a diabetic whose diet is good and who is receiving good treatment so that blood glucose is kept to near normal levels.

10.4 Treatment of Hyperlipoproteinaemia in Diabetes and Obesity

It is important to treat the obesity and diabetes to reduce the risk of cardiovascular disease as weight loss and improved metabolic control in diabetics will improve the lipoprotein profile.

Obesity

Weight loss through reduction in energy intake, is the most effective treatment of the obese, although weight loss in some obese people is difficult to achieve, may take several months and is not always sustained. There are some drugs which have been used, with some success, to help weight loss, notably the serotoninergic drugs such as fenfluramine, which potentiate the action of serotonin on the hypothalamus and give an increase in satiety. However fenfluramine has recently been removed from the market in US because of some unfavourable side effects. Surgical treatment, such as wiring the jaw, may be effective in the short tem, but weight is often regained once the wire is removed. Major surgery to reduce the size of the stomach or to by-pass part of the small intestine is usually restricted to treatment of the grossly obese in whom other treatments have failed.

Weight reduction is often accompanied by a reduction in total and LDL cholesterol. Although HDL cholesterol may fall while weight is being lost it usually is increased once a stable but lower weight is achieved. The general practitioner should monitor the overweight patient and recommend methods of weight loss and improved exercise regimes. He should provide health education for his patients, particularly parents, to prevent overeating and weight gain in children, so as to prevent obesity from developing and to reduce its progress if already present.

Diabetes

Careful diagnosis is required. IDDM patients have to be treated with daily insulin. In contrast dietary modification and exercise are the first recommendations for patients with NIDDM. If these fail to reduce the symptoms then hypoglycaemic drugs may be necessary. These have to be chosen carefully so that the hyperlipoproteinaemia is not made worse. Dietary advice has to be given on an individual basis if possible. For the obese diabetic weight loss is necessary and most beneficial so that energy restriction is required until a satisfactory lower weight is obtained. Diets should contain complex carbohydrate and avoid glucose or sucrose so that hyperglycaemic peaks can be prevented. Saturated fat should be reduced and monosaturated fat consumed in preference to reduce plasma cholesterol.

Two main groups of drugs are available to treat diabetes: the sulphonylureas and the biguanides, the former lower blood glucose by stimulating insulin release from the pancreas. They may also reduce the hepatic release of glucose and diminish insulin resistance. Tolbutamide is the mildest of these drugs and is well tolerated. Chlorpropamide is stronger and may produce hypoglycaemia, which can also be harmful. The more recent drug of this group, gliclazide is now widely used and has few side effects. The mechanism of action of the biguanides is uncertain but the biguanide, metformin increases insulin sensitivity and increases peripheral uptake of glucose. It acts synergistically with sulphonylureas so that dual drug treatment can be used for treatment of intractable diabetes.

Even if good metabolic control is achieved with respect to plasma glucose, hyperlipoproteinaemia may persist and hypolipidaemic drugs may be necessary.

Treatment of hyperlipoproteinaemia in diabetes

Lipid lowering drugs were described in chapter 5. Some but not all of these can be used to reduce the hyperlipoproteinaemia of diabetics. Nicotinic acid should be avoided as it impairs glycaemic control. Fibric acids that can be used to treat severe hypertriglyceridaemia in diabetes must be avoided in patients with diabetic nephropathy. Bile acid sequestrants are effective in lowering LDL cholesterol in some patients with NIDDM, but as they can raise plasma TAG they cannot be used in subjects with hypertriglyceridaemia. The main hypolipidaemic drugs for treatment of diabetics, except for patients with hyperchylomicronaemia, are the HMGCoA reductase inhibitors, the statins. These drugs which reduce cholesterol biosynthesis increase LDL receptor expression and increase LDL and VLDL remnant clearance from the blood. They are well tolerated and do not interfere with the control of hyperglycaemia. Combination of statins with bile acid sequestrants is possible but the effect of these drugs on the patient's metabolism and health must be carefully monitored.

10.5 Conclusion

Since it is now well established and well perceived that obesity and diabetes are two diseases in which the risk of developing cardiovascular disease is much increased, there is growing concern in the medical profession to treat those who suffer from these metabolic disorders as early as possible. Early diagnosis is therefore essential. Treatment of the underlying metabolic disease as well as the accompanying hyperlipoproteinaemia will help to improve the prognosis and prevent the severity of coronary heart disease and other symptoms of atherosclerosis.

Key references

General

Bjorntorp, P. and Brodoff, B.N. (eds) (1992) Obesity. J.B.Lippincott Co.

The origins and consequences of obesity (1996) Ciba Foundation Symposium 201. John Wiley & Sons

Moller, D.E. ed. (1993) Insulin Resistance. John Wiley & Sons

Obesity

Manson, J.E. *et al.* (1995) Body weight and mortality among women. New England Journal of Medicine 333, 677-685

Willett, W.C. *et al.* (1995) Weight, weight change and coronary heart disease in women. Journal of the American Medical Association 273, 461-465

Blum, W.F. *et al.* (1998) Human and clinical perspectives on leptin. Proceedings of the Nutrition Society 57, 477-485

Action of Insulin

Moule, S.K. and Denton, R.M. (1997) Multiple signalling pathways involved in the metabolic effects of insulin. American Journal of Cardiology 80 (3A) 41A-49A

Shepherd, P.R., Withers, D.J. and Siddle, K. (1998) Phosphoinositide 3-kinase: the key switch mechanism in insulin signalling. Biochemical Journal 333, 471-490

Insulin resistance in obesity and in diabetes

Nolan, J.J. *et al.* (1997) Mechanisms of the kinetic defect in insulin action in obesity and NIDDM. Diabetes 46, 994-1000

Obesity and atherosclerosis

Kortelainen, M. and Sarkioja, T. (1997) Extent and composition of coronary lesion and degree of cardiac hypertrophy in relation to abdominal fatness in men under 40 years of age. Arteriosclerosis Thrombosis & Vascular Biology 17, 574-579

Sniderman, A.D. *et al.* (1998) The adipocyte, fatty acid trapping and atherogenesis. Arteriosclerosis, Thrombosis and Vascular Biology 18, 147-151

Insulin Dependent Diabetes Mellitus (IDDM)

Gottlieb, P.A. and Eisenbarth, G.S. (1998) Diagnosis and treatment of pre-insulin dependent diabetes. Annual Reviews of Medicine 49, 391-405

Non Insulin Dependent Diabetes (NIDDM)

Terauchi, Y. *et al.* (1997) Development of non-insulin-dependent diabetes mellitus in the double knockout mice with disruption of insulin receptor substrate-1 and b-cell glucokinase genes. Journal of Clinical Investigation 99, 861-866

Diabetes and Atherosclerosis

Turner, R.C. *et al.* (1998) Risk factors for coronary artery disease in non-insulin dependent diabetes mellitus: United Kingdom prospective diabetes study (UKPDS:23). British Medical Journal.316, 823-828

Laakso, M. and Lehto, S. (1998) Epidemiology of risk factors for cardiovascular disease in diabetes and impaired glucose tolerance. Atherosclerosis 137, S65-S73

Treatment of Hyperlioproteinaemia in Diabetes and Obesity

Garg, A. (1998) Treatment of diabetic dyslipidemia. American Journal of Cardiology 81(4A) 47B-51B

Schwartz, M.W. and Brunzell, J.D. (1997) Regulation of body adiposity and the problem of obesity. Arteriosclerosis Thrombosis & Vascular Biology 17, 233-238

11 Prevention and Regression of Atherosclerosis

11.1 Introduction

There are a number of dietary measures that can be taken to prevent or reduce the risk of the development of atherosclerosis. Once clinical symptoms of atherosclerosis are manifest in an individual there are various treatments possible which differ in their mechanism of action and efficacy: these will be discussed below. In some cases the reduction in size of atherosclerotic lesions, and therefore reduction in risk of these lesions giving rise to medical problems, is possible. This process of **regression** has been observed but, like the progression of the disease, may be a slow process in man. The treatment of atherosclerosis will be discussed first, below, and then prevention of the disease will be considered.

11.2 Treatment of clinically manifest atherosclerosis and the regression of atherosclerosis

Treatment of clinical symptoms of atherosclerosis

Treatment has to be on an individual basis dependent on the medical symptoms and diagnosis. The use of thrombolytic drugs is usually necessary for myocardial infarct and stroke to prevent immediate recurrence and to aid dispersal of the thrombi that have caused symptoms. Medical treatment, by drugs or surgery, may be required to restore the oxygen supply to the tissue made ischaemic by the stenosis. Once the initial clinical condition has stabilised the patient may be put on a strict diet or drug regime or a combination of both a diet and drug programme to reduce the risk factor(s) present in the individual in order to prevent further progression of the underlying atherosclerosis and to provide conditions that may favour regression of exsisting lesions.

Lesions most likely to cause medical symptoms

The ultrastructure and chemical composition of atherosclerotic lesions varies as the lesions develop and progress in size and complexity (see chapter 2). Some of these lesions are more vulnerable to rupture and it is these more "unstable lesions" which will give rise to clinical symptoms such as angina and myocardial infarct.

The nature of atheroma in the coronary arteries that make them vulnerable to rupture and thus potential sites for thrombus formation has been examined. The unstable lesions have a higher content of lipid and only a thin fibrous cap whereas those lesions with more smooth muscle cells, collagen-rich extracellular matrix and little lipid tend to be more stable. The region of rupture of a vulnerable lesion often has many active macrophage foam cells. It is believed that the metalloproteinases secreted by these cells renders the extracellular matrix less stable. This and the soft core of extracellular lipid in the lesion makes the lesion susceptible to fissure formation and plaque rupture. The latter may be precipitated by mechanical or hemodynamic forces.

The substance which initiates the formation of a thrombus when a lesion is ruptured is known as tissue factor. This has been identified, immunohistochemically, in foam cells and in the extracellular lipid core of atherosclerotic lesions. Initially platelets aggregate over the rupture and then as coagulation progresses the platelets become enmeshed in fibrin and if erythroctes become caught in the growing thrombus a red thrombus forms which may grow in size sufficient to block or occlude the lumen of the artery.

In a particular individual there may be a variety of atherosclerotic lesions of different sizes and states of progression. It is, unfortunately, not possible to predict which lesions will give rise to clinical symptoms. If the rupture of a plaque is sealed by a thrombus within the confines of the lesion and the wall of the artery (termed a mural thrombus) this may not give rise to clinical symptoms but the lesion will progress and the thrombus will be assimilated into the lesion. This modified lesion may give trouble in the future. If, however, the thrombus becomes sufficiently large to occlude the artery then clinical symptoms ensue. Transient occlusion can lead to angina and more prolonged occlusion to myocardial infarct or sudden coronary death. Consequently the rupture of vulnerable atheroma is potentially extremely dangerous and could be fatal.

Regression of atherosclerotic lesions

If those lesions which have a high lipid content are more susceptible to rupture if follows that reduction of lesion lipid content should reduce the risk of incidence of plaque rupture. It has been proposed that plasma lipid lowering treatment, in man, prevents clinical events of cardiovascular disease by causing selective regression of vulnerable lipid-rich atherosclerotic lesions. Evidence to support this hypothesis is discussed below.

It is possible to examine arteriograms before and after lipid lowering treatment, in man, and observe reopening of formerly obstructed arteries and a reduction in size of some lesions after treatment. The changes in size of lesions gives an approximate indication of the extent of progression and/or regression and thus indicates the efficacy of the treatment. However, the coronary arteriogram does not give details of lesion ultrastructure nor is it possible to examine this in a live person. The ultrastructure of human atherosclerotic lesions has been determined from examination of post mortem arteries (see chapter 2). In the early lesions, lipid is mainly intracellular in macrophage foam cells. In more advanced lesions, lipid is extracellular and forms a core at the base of the lesion. In atheroma, the lipid may comprise as much as 60% of the dry weight. Most of the lipid is cholesterol, mainly present as cholesterol ester though free cholesterol is also present. Free cholesterol can be accommodated in phospholipid membranes but when it's concentration exceeds the capacity of the membrane to dissolve cholesterol, the cholesterol begins to crystallise. Cholesterol monohydrate crystals are found in atheromatous lesions, usually near the base of the lesion. It has been suggested that growth of these crystals in lysosomes may cause rupture of the lysosomes, release of lysosomal hydrolytic enzymes, contributing to cell death and the development of the necrotic core of the lesion. During regression, cholesterol ester is first hydrolysed and mobilised out of the lesion. Macrophages foam cells also disappear from the lesions. The cholesterol monohydrate crystals, which are almost inert, take a long time to disappear. With the exception of elastin, the extracellular matrix material and calcium deposits which have accumulated in the atherosclerotic lesion during it's development and progression probably do not diminish during the process of regression. Regression of atheroma in the aorta (induced in male rhesus monkeys by feeding a high saturated fat and high cholesterol diet, for approximately five years) has been seen after feeding a cholesterol-free diet for a further four years. Regression also occurred in the atherosclerotic lesions of the coronary and carotid arteries of these monkeys and was characterised by a reduction in size and lipid content of the lesions.

Effect of lipid lowering treatment on the regression of atherosclerotic lesions

A review of the results of sixteen randomised trials, in which the effects of lipid lowering treatment was determined by examining coronary arteriograms, in patients with elevated plasma cholesterol and evidence of coronary heart disease, showed both reduction in progression and regression of atherosclerotic lesions was possible. A variety of lipid lowering regimes were employed but in each trial the effective lowering of plasma cholesterol was accompanied by a reduction in size of some lesions as judged from the arteriograms, but more importantly, there was a reduction in the number of clinical events of cardiovascular disease. It was suggested that the reduction of clinical events was most probably due to plaque stabilisation.

The results of some of the clinical trials in which the progression or regression of lesions was monitored, by measuring coronary lumen size on the arteriograms before and after treatment, are summarised in table 11.1.

Many studies have shown that, in man, plasma cholesterol concentration and specifically LDL cholesterol can be lowered by modification of diet (see section 11.3). More dramatic decreases in plasma LDL cholesterol can be achieved by certain drugs or surgical treatment. The clinical trials recorded in table 1 show that the reduction of LDL cholesterol may be accompanied by a reduced rate of progression and in some patients a regression of atherosclerotic lesion as assessed by the size of the lesions measured with the coronary arteriograms. Some of the treatments also increased HDL cholesterol which may have contributed to the improvements seen in the treated groups.

Treatment to reduce other risk factors

As described in chapter 10, the treatment of obesity by weight loss and the amelioration of the symptoms of diabetes can reduce the risk of cardiovascular disease. Part of this reduced risk may be the modification of the lipoprotein profile to one which is less likely to cause atherosclerosis or less likely to enhance the progression of atherosclerosis if it is already established.

High blood pressure and an addiction to smoking in patients who already have coronary artery disease compound the risk of further, potentially fatal clinical symptoms and these patients must be treated to reduce high blood pressure and advised to stop smoking. Although these two risk factors do not necessarily modify the lipoprotein profile they do affect lipoprotein metabolism. Thus high blood pressure may increase the extent to which LDL enters the intima of the artery wall and smoking increases the susceptibility of LDL to oxidation: both these processes may facilitate the development and progression of atherosclerosis. Reduction of elevated blood pressure and cessation of smoking can improve the prognosis of patients with coronary heart disease.

11.3 Prevention of Atherosclerosis

While it may not be possible to prevent atherosclerosis developing in people with a strong genetic predisposition for the disease, it is possible to reduce the risks and to reduce the numbers who will show clinical symptoms of the disease in the general population.

In chapters 7-9 we have already discussed the potential effects of various macro- and micro-nutrients on liporotein metabolism. The present

Table 11.1 The effect of lipid lowering treatment on the progression and regression of atherosclerosis and the incidence of clinical events after treatment.

*Trial no.**	*Treatment of test group (Number of patients/ number of years of treatment)*	*% fall of LDL*	*% of patients showing progression control/test*	*% of patients showing regression control/test*	*% of patients with clinical events of cardio- vascular disease control/test*
1	Cholestyramine (116/5)	26	49/32	9.6/12.2	8.4/5.6 (death or myocardial infarct)
2	Partial ileal bypass surgery (838/10)	37.7	65.4/37.5 (5yr)	4.7/12.6	30/20 (death or myocardial infarct)
3	a)Lovastatin +colestipol b) Niacin + colestipol (120/2.5)	46 32	46/21 46/25	11/32 11/39	19.2/6.5 19.2/4.2 (death or myocardial infarct or surgery)
4	a) Diet b) Diet + cholestyramine (74/3.25)	16 36	46/15 46/12	4/38 4/33	36/11 36/4 (cardio- vascular events)
5	Lovastatin (270/2)	38	33/23.6	9.7/17.9	25/17.9 (death, myocardial infarct, surgery or angina)
6	Lovastatin (331/2)	29	50/33	13/19	13.6/9.7 (death, myocardial infarct or angina)
7	Simvastatin (381/4)	31	30.3/24.6	11.2/19.8	27/20.7 (cardio- vascular events)
8	Pravastatin (885/2)	29	54.8/44	9/16.7	28/18.3 (death, myocardial infarct, surgery or angina)

(*Trials reported in table 1 (References for these studies cited by Maher (1995).

1. National heart, lung and blood institute type II coronary intervention study
2. Program on the surgical control of the hyperlipidemias (POSCH)
3. Familial Atherosclerosis study (FATS)
4. St Thomas Atherosclerosis study (STARS)
5. The monitored atherosclerosis regression study (MARS)
6. The Canadian coronary atherosclerosis intervention trial
7. The multicentre anti-atheroma study (MAAS)
8. The regression growth evaluation statin study (REGRESS)

section reviews the potential effects of specific diets, dietary recommendations and foods on lipoprotein metabolism and development of atherosclerosis.

Specific national dietary recommendations

In USA the National Cholesterol Education Programme, NCEP, was established in 1980. The dietary recommendations for the general population of the NCEP "step 1" diet was to lower fat to less than 30% of the total energy with saturated fat less than 10% of total energy and cholesterol less than 300mg/day. For those whose lipids did not fall sufficiently with this diet, a "step 2" diet was recommended in which saturated fat was reduced to less than 7% and cholesterol to less than 200mg/day. Compared with a baseline diet of 35-40% energy as fat and 13-16% as saturated fat, the "step 2" diet was found to reduce LDL cholesterol by 19% and HDL cholesterol by 17% in men but there was a large individual variability in response to the diet. Despite this variability, there has been a marked improvement in the mortality figures from coronary and other cardiovascular diseases in the USA which in part may be attributed to improved diet, and also to improved coronary and general health care, improved hospital care and the use of thrombolytic drugs.

There have been guidelines proposed by other expert committees with similar recommendations. The British Hyperlipidemia Association advocated a reduction of dietary fat to less than 30% and saturated fat to less than 10% of the total energy intake. The British Cardiac Society recommended these figures, for the general population be less than 35% and less than 15% while the European Atherosclerosis Society (EAS) recommended values similar to the British Hyperlipidaemia Association and NCEP with an additional recommendation of less than 10% polyunsaturated fat and less than 10% monounsaturated fat. The EAS also suggested a "step 2" diet with less than 25% fat and less than 150mg cholesterol/day. The UK Department of Health, Committee on Medical Aspects of Food Policy, 1994 Guidelines have already been discussed in chapter 8. In addition to the macronutrient recommendations described, they also translate this nutrient data into food consumption data (table 11.2).

Mediterannean diet, Cretan diet

In the 1960s it was observed that the mortality from coronary heart disease in Southern Europe, the Mediterranean countries, was 2-3 fold lower than in Northern Europe or USA. Within Southern Europe the mortality figures for Crete were particularly low. At that time the diet in Crete was rich in legumes, fruit and olive oil with less meat than other Mediteranean countries, and contained a moderate amount of fish

Table 11.2 Food recommendations for reducing cardiovascular disease*

Food	Recommendation
Fish	Two portions per week one of which is oily fish
Fat spreads and dairy produce	Use reduced fat rather than full fat products
Fats and oils	Replace fats rich in saturated fatty acids with those rich in monounsaturated fatty acids
Fruit and vegetables	Increase consumption of vegetables, fruit, potatoes and bread by at least 50%

*Taken from: Department of Health. Report on Health and Social Subjects 46 Nutritional Aspects of Cardiovascular Disease (1994) Report of the Cardiovascular Review Group, Committee on Medical Aspects of Food Policy (London, HMSO)

and red wine. In the Lyon intervention trial an adapted Cretan diet was compared with a prudent diet for the treatment of patients recovering from myocardial infarction. While plasma cholesterol and LDL cholesterol were similar on the two diets, the Cretan diet gave a better protection against subsequent cardiovascular clinical events. The simulated Cretan diet contained significantly more linolenic acid and less linoleic acid and it has been suggested that this ratio of linolenic acid to linoleic acid may be antithrombogenic. In addition the Cretan diet had a high concentration of natural antioxidants which may protect against the development and further progression of atherosclerosis.

The French Paradox

The difference in consumption of vegetables and plant oils in the diet may explain the paradox that there are some countries with similar levels of plasma cholesterol and saturated fat intake that have large differences in coronary mortality. Thus, for example, Finland and Scotland have a significantly lower consumption of vegetables and a dramatically higher coronary mortality compared with France despite similar cholesterol levels and high saturated fat intake in the three countries. The paradox may be explained by the high antioxidant content of the plant materials preventing the development, and/ or reducing the rate of progression, of atherosclerosis.

This phenomenon of great differences in coronary mortality despite similarities in plasma cholesterol levels and saturated fat intake is often referred to as the French Paradox and attributed in part to the consumption of red wine in France and other Mediterranean countries with low mortalities from cardiovascular disease. Red wine contains flavonoids which inhibit LDL oxidation *in vitro* (see chapter 9).

Whilst dietary antioxidants such as vitamin E and vitamin C do not produce lowering of plasma lipids, they do appear to reduce the risk of cardiovascular disease. In view of the possible protection of LDL against oxidation, *in vivo*, (see chapter 9) the antioxidant vitamins may be antiatherogenic and therefore comprise an important and essential component of a healthy diet. Other dietary components with potential antioxidant properties, such as the flavonoids and polyphenols, may also be important in offering protection against the development and / or progression of atherosclerosis.

Functional foods

The term functional food has been used to describe food products which are marketed on the basis of an implied health benefit. In many countries the claims that can be made relating to the beneficial effects of foods are closely regulated. Thus, it is unlikely that a product could be marketed in the UK with a claim that it, "prevents you from developing heart disease". However, a claim such as, "may help to reduce plasma cholesterol as part of a low fat diet", may be acceptable. Functional foods can be divided into three major classes; those which are established parts of our diet which have subsequently been found to have beneficial effects, those which are formulated using established food ingredient in order to try and impart specific health benefits and finally those which include novel ingredients which are believed to impart specific health benefits. Some examples of each type of Functional Food are listed in table 11.3. In the rest of this section we will concentrate on foods that have been developed using novel ingredients and designed specifically to try and influence lipoprotein metabolism.

Table 11.3 Some examples of functional foods

Food	*Active components*
Traditional Foods	
Olive Oil	Oleic acid, antioxidants
Porridge	Soluble fibre
Foods formulated with traditional ingredients	
Margarines & low fat spreads	Unsaturated fatty acids, vitamin E
Foods using new ingredients	
Fermented milk products	"Live" bacterial cultures
Fat replacers	Starch, protein (modified to resemble some properties of fat) sucrose polyesters
Plant sterol enriched margarine	Sitastanol ester

Fermented milk products

For many years it has been suggested that foods containing fermented milk may have specific cholesterol -lowering properties. These claims appear to have their origin in studies carried out in Africa on Masia Tribesmen. Despite consuming diets rich in cholesterol and saturated fat, these people were found to have a very low incidence of cardiovascular disease. One common part of their diet was large amounts of fermented milk. This led to a series of studies in which Western subjects were asked to consume large amounts of yoghurt which yielded mixed results in terms of cholesterol lowering. More recently a number of yoghurts have become commercially available and claim to have specific cholesterol-reducing properties. The apparent "active" ingredient appears to be the type of culture with which the milk is fermented. It is claimed that organisms within the yoghurt colonize the gastrointestinal tract and in some way impart a cholesterol-lowering effect. The mechanisms whereby such "probiotics" exert their effects remains to be established. Some, but not all of these products, have been demonstrated to have specific effects in well-controlled scientific studies. However, as yet results appear to be rather inconsistent between studies, suggesting that the effects may be strongly related to individual characteristics, such as dietary habits, of the population studied. An alternative strategy is to include within a food product a substance, such as different types of dietary fibre, which may enhance the growth of specific beneficial bacteria within the gastrointestinal tract. Such "prebiotics" have also been included in specific fermented milk products.

Fat replacers

A fat replacer can be defined as a food ingredient or technology which results in the replacement of fat in a food without sacrificing the organoleptic properties of the food. They can be further divided into **fat mimetics** and **fat substitutes**. The former are designed to fulfil some of the properties of fat in food such as "mouth feel" body and bulk but are not designed to replace fat on a gram for gram basis. These include starch-based products, those based on cellulose and/or gums, and microparticulated protein. On the other hand, fat substitutes resemble triacylglycerols in physical and chemical properties and can theoretically replace fat on a gram for gram basis. One of the most recent fat replacers to come on to the market is the mixture of **sucrose polyesters** known as "Olestra". This consists of a sucrose molecule to which are esterified six, seven or eight fatty acid molecules. This molecule is too big to be hydrolyzed by intestinal lipase and as a result none of the fatty acids are absorbed. Thus, while it may impart on food all the properties of fat, it yeilds no energy and no fatty acids to the body. While some concern has been expressed over possible detrimental effects on the absorption of lipid-soluble vitamins and over possible gastrointestinal side-effects of increasing the faecal fat load, Olestra is now used in a limited way in foods in the United States. Do these products have potential for cholesterol-lowering? The answer to this obviously depends on what is replaced in the diet. If fat-replacers are used to replace predominantly saturated fatty acid then they will have potential benefits. However, if these products simply replace mono- and/or poly-unsaturated fatty acids, in margarines for example, they might actually have a modest cholesterol-raising effect. Probably the most important role for these ingredients is in helping to reduce overall energy intake in the obese.

Plant sterols

Plants produce virtually no cholesterol but do produce a range of related sterols. Plant sterols such as sitosterol, stigmasterol and campesterol are present in the diet at similar concentrations to cholesterol itself. It has been known for many years that plant sterols have the ability to inhibit the absorption of cholesterol from the small intestine and thereby reduce plasma cholesterol. However, the magnitude of the effect is relatively small. More recently a sitosterol derivative, **sitastanol**, has been shown to be more potent in reducing plasma cholesterol. This has now been incorporated into margarine following transesterification with rape seed oil. At a daily intake of sitostanol of about 2g/day, the sitastanol ester-containing margarine has been shown to reduce plasma LDL cholesterol by about 14%. The margarine appears to well tolerated, sitastanol itself is not absorbed and does not appear to interfere with the absorption of fat-soluble vitamins. This functional food appears to offer a real possibility for wide-spread cholesterol-lowering on a population basis.

Weight loss

An analysis of seventy studies, in which weight reduction was monitored and lipoproteins measured, has shown that weight reduction is accompanied by a decrease in total plasma cholesterol and LDL cholesterol and triacylglycerol. The HDL cholesterol decreases while subjects are actively losing weight but increases again when weight reduction is maintained. The improvement in the lipoprotein profile after weight loss shows that this is an important way in which the risk of developing cardiovascular disease may be reduced in those who are overweight.

Drug treatment

For those people who are at a high risk of developing coronary heart disease, and who have a high plasma cholesterol which does not respond to dietary lowering or who are unable to adhere to a strict diet, it may be necessary to use drugs. A number of drugs are available which have been used effectively to treat hyperlipidaemias (see chapter 5). Plasma cholesterol lowering can be achieved with fibrates, niacin, bile acid sequestrants and HMGCoA reductase inhibitors, or a combination of these drugs. Hypercholesterolaemia in patients who already show symptoms of coronary heart disease can be reduced by drug treatment and the number of subsequent clinical symptoms reduced by these cholesterol lowering drugs, as shown in table 11.1. In some of these studies drug treatment accompanied dietary changes to improve the lipoprotein profile and the clinical outcome. High cholesterol levels in non-insulin dependent diabetics were effectively lowered by a combination of statin and sitostanol margarine.

As described in chapter 3, in the West of Scotland Study, the drug Pravastatin given to middle aged men with moderate hypercholesterolaemia (mean plasma cholesterol 7.0±0.6mM) but with no history of myocardial infarction reduced the incidence of myocardial infarct and death from cardiovascular disease. It is likely that these men already had incipient atherosclerosis. The drug treatment, by lowering the plasma cholesterol and LDL cholesterol (by 20% and 26% respectively) probably reduced the development and slowed the progression of atherosclerosis and thereby reducing the incidence of clinical events through stabilisation of atheromatous plaques and the reduced number of plaque rupture. This study provided support for the widespread use of drug treatment, for people with elevated plasma cholesterol, as preventative medicine.

Hormone Replacement therapy

It is well established that before menopause women are protected from atherosclerotic vascular disease compared to men and that after menopause risk substantially increases (Chapter 3). Considerable evidence exist to suggests that **hormone replacement therapy (HRT)** can reduces risk in postmenopausal women. **Oestrogen** administration to postmenopausal women appears to reduce plasma total and LDL cholesterol and increase HDL cholesterol. As a result HRT can be considered as a treatment in women with multiple risk factors for cardiovascular disease.

11.4 Conclusion

The prevention of atherosclerosis, and it's medical consequences is possible in many of the general population if sensible healthy diets and lifestyles are adopted from an early age. Some people may have, through their genetic makeup, or acquire, through unwise eating habits or lifestyle, one or more of the conditions known to be risk factors for developing coronary heart disease: eg. high plasma cholesterol, high blood pressure or smoking. If these conditions are minimised the risk of developing clinical symptoms of coronary heart disease can be reduced.

The term primary prevention with respect to coronary heart disease is used for strategies to reduce the risk factors in the general population and those at high risk but who do not have overt clinical symptoms eg. diabetics, patients with high cholesterol or high blood pressure or with a family history of coronary heart disease. As atherosclerosis is quite likely to be well advanced in these "high risk" people it might be more appropriate to term treatment in this group secondary prevention. The latter term is usually used for measures to prevent further occurrence of clinical events in those who already have some of the clinical symptoms of atherosclerotic disease.

As there is strong evidence that hypercholesterolaemia is associated with increased risk of coronary heart disease it is extremely important to impress on the population that a healthy diet, avoiding excess saturated fat, will reduce the risk of developing this disease. General practitioners and health workers need to be aware of the risk factors and the appropriate treatment to remove or minimise the conditions in their patients that might predispose to the development and progression of atherosclerosis and of the medical consequences. The health team should be able to advise or counsel their patients, where necessary, to change their eating habits, or adopt a more healthy lifestyle or to undergo lipid lowering treatment.

High plasma cholesterol concentrations can be lowered by reducing the quantity of saturated fat in the diet, by various drugs and by a combination of dietary and drug regimes. In order to ensure regression of atherosclerosis already present, these regimes have to be continued for long periods. To prevent the development of atherosclerosis and the progression of atherosclerotic lesions to give clinical symptoms of cardiovascular disease, protective diets should be in place from an early age, they must be continued through life and other risk factors should be avoided.

Key references

Lesions most likely to cause medical symptoms

Schroeder, A.P. and Falk, E. (1995) Vulnerable and dangerous coronary plaques. Atherosclerosis 118, S141-S149

Regression of atherosclerotic lesions

Brown, B.G. *et al*. (1993) Arteriographic view of treatment to achieve regression of coronary atherosclerosis and to prevent plaque disruption and clinical cardiovascular events. British Heart Journal 69. S48-S53

Small, D.M. (1998) Progression and regression of atherosclerotic lesions. Arteriosclerosis 8, 103-129

Strong, J.P. *et al.* (1994) Long term induction and regression of diet induced atherosclerotic lesions in rhesus monkeys. 1. Morphological and chemical evidence for regression of lesions in the aorta and carotid and peripheral arteries. Arteriosclerosis and Thrombosis 14, 958-964

Clinical trials to assess regression

Maher, V.M.G. (1995) Coronary atherosclerosis stabilisation: an achievable goal. Atherosclerosis 118, S91-S101

Specific dietary recommendations

Schaefer, E.J. *et al.* (1997) Individual variability in lipoprotein response to the National Cholesterol Education Programme step 2 diets. American Journal of Clinical Nutrition. 65, 823-830

Cobbe, S.M. and Shepherd, J. (1993) Cholesterol reduction in the prevention of coronary heart disease: therapeutic rationale and guidelines. British Heart Journal 69, S63-S69

Cretan Diet

Renaud, S. *et al.* (1995) Cretan Meditarranean diet for the prevention of coronary heart disease. American Journal of Clinical Nutrition 61, 1360S-1367S

The French Paradox

Artauld-Wild, S. *et al.* (1993) Differences in coronary mortality can be explained by differences in cholesterol and saturated fat intakes in 40 countries but not in France and Finland. Circulation 88, 2771-2779

Weight loss

Lichtenstein, A.H. *et al.* (1994) Short term consumption of a low fat diet beneficially affects plasma lipid concentrations only when accompanied by weight loss. Arteriosclerosis and Thrombosis 14, 1751-1760

Dattilo, A.M. and Kris-Etherton, P.M. (1992) Effects of weight reduction on blood lipids and lipoproteins: a meta-analysis. American Journal of Clinical Nutrition 56, 320-328

Drugs for lowering plasma cholesterol

Gylling, H. and Miettinen, T.A. (1996) Effects of inhibiting cholesterol absorption and synthesis on cholesterol and lipoprotein metabolism in hypercholesterolemic non-insulin-dependent diabetic men. Journal of Lipid Research 37, 1776-1785

Shepherd, J. *et al.* (1995) Prevention of coronary heart disease with pravastatin in men with hypecholesterolemia. New England Journal of Medicine 333, 1301-1307

Functional Foods

Hornstra, G. *et al.* (1998) Functional food science and the cardiovascular system. British Journal of Nutrition 80(Supplement 1) S113-S146

Index